Hildegard of Bingen's
Spiritual Remedies

Hildegard of Bingen's Spiritual Remedies

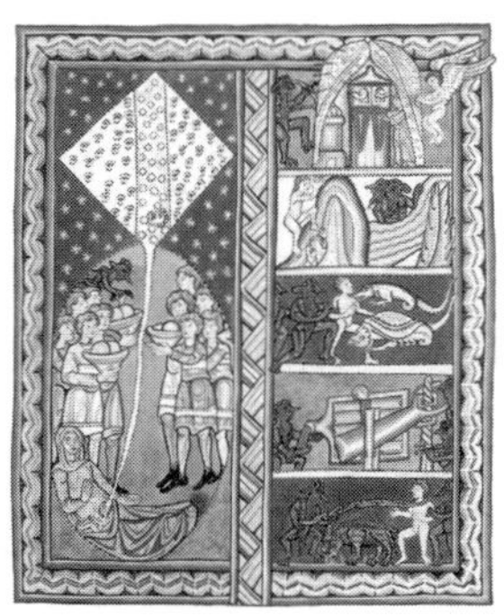

Dr. Wighard Strehlow

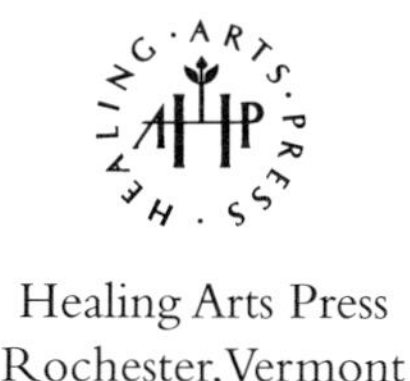

Healing Arts Press
Rochester, Vermont

Healing Arts Press
One Park Street
Rochester, Vermont 05767
www.InnerTraditions.com

Healing Arts Press is a division of Inner Traditions International

Library of Congress Cataloging-in-Publication Data

Strehlow, Wighard
Hildegard of Bingen's spiritual remedies / Wighard Strehlow.
p. cm.
Includes bibliographical references and index.
ISBN 0-89281-985-5
1. Spiritual healing. 2. Alternative medicine. 3. Hildegard, Saint, 1098–1179. I. Title.
BT732.5 .S87 2002
615.8—dc21
2002017125

Printed and bound in the United States at Capital City Press

10 9 8 7 6 5 4 3 2 1

Text design and layout by Rachel Goldenberg

This book was typeset in Bembo with Snell Roundhand as the display typeface

To my wife, Karin,

and my four children, George, Stefanie, Sofia, and Harry.

Thank you for your love and spirit.

CONTENTS

Prologue A SPIRITUAL GUIDE THROUGH THE THIRD MILLENNIUM WITH HILDEGARD OF BINGEN xi

Do We Need a New Medicine?

Introduction THE POWER OF SPIRITUAL FITNESS 1

Virtues and Vices

Turning the Evil into the Virtuous

The Healing Power of Precious Stones and Crystals

Chapter 1 PRINCIPLES OF HILDEGARD'S PSYCHOTHERAPY 12
The Cosmic and Divine Forces of the Human Soul

1. Vision: The Cosmic Dimension of Humanity

2. Vision: Humanity in the Rhythm of the Four Elements

3. Vision: Relationship between Body and Soul

4. Vision: The Trinity in the Unity

Chapter 2 SPIRITUALITY AND HEALING 38

Is There a World Ethos?

Discovery of Cosmic Psychosomatic Values

Practical Application of Hildegard's Psychotherapy

Liber Vitae Meritorum (The Book of Virtues and Vices)

Our Social Relationship

Self-analysis

Rediscovery of Hildegard's Psychotherapy

Healing Is a Multidimensional Process

Friendship with the Angels

The Cosmic Christ and the Power of Love

Anatomy of the Human Body and Soul

The Language of the Soul

The Autonomic Nervous System: Bridge between Body and Soul

Ordo Virtutum: The Dance of Life with Virtues and Vices

Chapter 3 THE EASTMAN 60

The First Seven Powers and the Seven Senses

1. *Amor saeculi* and *Amor caelestis* • Material Love and Heavenly Love

2. *Petulantia* and *Disciplina* • Petulance and Discipline

3. *Joculatrix* and *Verecundia* • Love of Entertainment and Love of Simplicity

4. *Obduratio* and *Misericordia* • Hard-heartedness and Compassion

5. *Ignavia* and *Divina victoria* • Cowardice and God's Victory

6. *Ira* and *Patientia* • Anger and Tranquillity

7. *Inepta laetitia* and *Gemitus ad Deum* • Inappropriate Mirth and Yearning for God

Chapter 4 THE WESTMAN 107

8. *Ingluvies ventri* and *Abstinentia* • Gluttony and Abstinence

9. *Acerbitas* and *Vera largitas* • Bitterness of Heart and Generosity

10. *Impietas* and *Pietas* • Wickedness and Devotion

11. *Fallacitas* and *Veritas* • Lying and Truth

12. *Contentio* and *Pax* • Contention and Peace

13. *Infelicitas* and *Beatitudo* • Unhappiness and Blessedness

14. *Immoderatio* and *Discretio* • Immoderation and Discretion

15. *Perditio animarum* and *Salvatio animarum* • Lost Soul and Saved Soul

Chapter 5 THE NORTHMAN 137

Infancy: The Third Section from Hip to Knee

The Acquired Virtues of Childhood

16. *Superbia* and *Humilitas* • Arrogance and Humility

17. *Invidia* and *Charitas* • Envy and Charity

18. *Inanis gloria* and *Timor Domini* • Thirst for Glory and Reverence for God

19. *Inobedientia* and *Obedientia* • Disobedience and Obedience

20. *Infidelitas* and *Fides* • Lack of Faith and Faith

21. *Desperatio* and *Spes* • Despair and Hope

22. *Luxuria* and *Castitas* • Obscenity and Chastity

Chapter 6 THE SOUTHMAN 168

23. *Injustitia* and *Justitia* • Injustice and Justice

24. *Torpor* and *Fortitudo* • Lethargy and Fortitude

25. *Oblivio* and *Sanctitas* • Oblivion and Holiness

26. *Inconstantia* and *Constantia* • Instability and Stability

27. *Cura terrenorum* and *Caeleste desiderium* • Concern for Worldly Goods and Heavenly Desire

28. *Obstinatio* and *Compunctio cordis* • Obstinacy and Remorse

29. *Cupiditas* and *Contemptus mundi* • Craving and Letting Go

30. *Discordia* and *Concordia* • Discord and Concord

Chapter 7 The New Elders Ascend to the Summit 208

The Supreme Allroundman

31. *Scurrilitas* and *Reverentia* • Scurrility and Reverence

32. *Vagatio* and *Stabilitas* • Vagabondage and Stability

33. *Maleficium* and *Cultus Dei* • Occultism and Dedication to God

34. *Avaritia* and *Sufficientia* • Avarice and Satisfaction

35. *Tristitia* and *Caeleste gaudium* • Melancholy and Heavenly Joy

Chapter 8 Fasting: Discover Your Real Personality 244

Long-term Fasting

Bread Fasting

Hard-core Fasting

Bibliography 252

Index 253

About Hildegard of Bingen 258

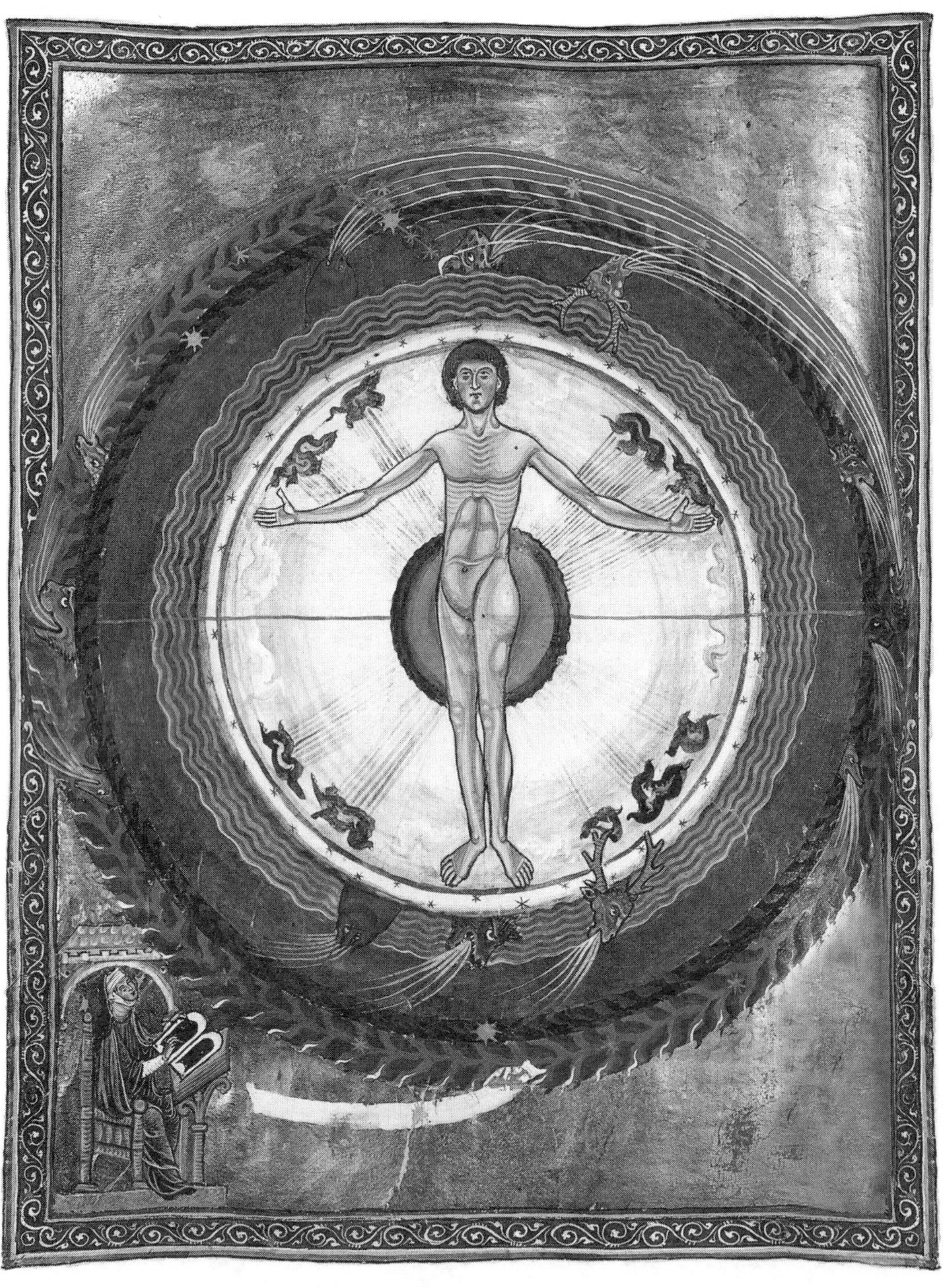

Humanity in the Center of the Universe. You are the center of the universe, spiritually created in the image and likeness of God himself (LDO, Vision 3)

Prologue
A Spiritual Guide through the Third Millennium with Hildegard of Bingen

Some 850 years ago Hildegard of Bingen described in her visionary study of cosmic psychotherapy, the Book of Values in Life, thirty-five risk factors that can destroy humanity and life on earth, along with the thirty-five healing forces counteracting this possible catastrophe. Hildegard of Bingen, a Benedictine abbess, was admired as *prophetissa teutonica* (German prophet) by her contemporaries. In her visionary illuminations we see that everything is inseparably connected in the cosmic web of the universe. We also see that all our deeds have a cosmic impact, either life-restoring or life-destroying. The universe is the target of our doing and reflects back the positive or negative energy onto all creatures.

Hildegard foresees a time when the universe will have to heal itself by way of natural catastrophes, because humanity has damaged and polluted the four life elements—fire, air, water, and the earth. We are now actually very clearly witnessing cosmic healing in the form of tornadoes, earthquakes, and flooding as a result of our progress-at-any-price mentality in Western society. Today's ecological collapse is the helplessness of our Western rationalism to understand life and the universe as *one.* In contrast to the mystical wisdom and knowledge of the East, Western science has in the past few centuries abandoned any spiritual dimension and is responsible for the environmental disasters plaguing this fragile planet. The growing awareness of nuclear and ecological threats to continued human existence brings into focus Hildegard's visions of God the Creator and the working of the universe as a unity. Hildegard's wisdom can heal the split between science and spirituality because it provides a synthesis of science and nature with religion. The illuminations by Hildegard of Bingen show the soul's journey through life in harmony with nature and in harmony with God, which we must hope will become mainstream thinking in the West in this new millennium.

Do We Need a New Medicine?

The new killer sicknesses of Western society were more or less rare in the past, especially in the East and in native societies such as Native Americans in the United States and the Aborigines in central Australia. The ailments are mostly the result of bad nutrition, a stress-filled lifestyle, and the loss of a spiritual dimension in society as a whole. We call these civilization sicknesses autoaggressive, meaning we are killing ourselves.

There is a great gap between the progress of medical science in intensive-care treatment and the helplessness in regard to the modern autoaggressive diseases such as heart attack and stroke, cancer, and arthritis. These diseases are for the most part incurable because the underlying spiritual risk factors are fatalistically ignored by the medical profession: We do not know where these sicknesses come from; therefore, we do not have any healing remedies. We can only suppress these diseases with aggressive means—surgery, chemotherapy, and radiation. Cancer reflects the desperate condition of the human soul and it will, despite surgery, keep returning until the spiritual risk factor causing it is eliminated.

In her last visionary book, *Liber Divinorum Operum* (The Book on the Work of God), Hildegard opens our eyes to the four dimensions in which holistic healing occurs simultaneously:

- physical healing with natural remedies and nutrition
- healing with thirty-five spiritual healing forces of the soul

- healing with the power of the four cosmic elements
- restoration through "oneness" with God—the "at-one-ment" that brings holistic health

Hildegard of Bingen was one of the first to integrate natural and spiritual healing forces. Hildegard's synthesis of man and nature, cosmos and Creator, unites the best of the wisdom of our fathers and mothers to heal our meaningless and superficial modern society of its spiritual poverty.

Hildegard of Bingen's Spiritual Remedies summarizes Hildegard's spiritual principles from the following five visionary books:

Scivias (SC), or Know the Way of Healing, the book on cosmic medicine
Liber Divinorum Operum (LDO), her psychotherapeutic book
Liber Vitae Meritorum (LVM), a medicinal book
Causae et Curae (CC), medical textbook
Liber Simplicis Medicinae, the book of natural healing methods, or *Physica* (PH).

Considering the intricacy and richness of the universe and the interconnection of humanity and goodness, Hildegard illustrates difficult topics with crystal-clear images. Her books are packed with brilliant illuminations showing geometric projections of the complex world reduced to essential patterns. The meditations in *Hildegard of Bingen's Spiritual Remedies* are based on her artistic illuminations, functioning as a multimedia show that will open our eyes to the unity of religion and science.

INTRODUCTION

The Power of Spiritual Fitness

Today people all over the world experience health and well-being through physical fitness—sports, yoga, ta'i chi, kung fu, and dance, for example.

Spiritual fitness also helps us experience health and well-being. It opens the window to an inner power that connects us with the energy of the entire universe and can help us understand our own nature so that we can live richer, happier, and healthier lives.

With the help of this book, we will see that almost all sicknesses are caused by the malfunction of the human soul and a spiritual blackout of the inner personality. Instead of fighting against the misery and evil by cutting away the sicknesses with surgery, chemical treatment, and radiation, we will see that all symptoms contain the message that something positive is hiding behind the evil. Using the negative energy behind the evil, we will learn to transform it into good, sickness into health, weakness into strength, and our enemies into our friends.

The power of this spiritual wisdom reveals the beneficial relationship between body and soul. The soul, in fact, controls the function of the body, including the heart, digestion, sexuality, and the power of the immune system. We will see how thirty-five spiritual risk factors suppress the immune system and how thirty-five spiritual healing forces can improve and strengthen the entire body. Through the wisdom of Hildegard of Bingen's visionary work, we begin to understand the deeper nature of the human soul and its relationship with the human body, in particular the autonomic nervous system.

On the thirty-five vertebrae of the spinal cord, we can trace the thirty-five spiritual forces of the human soul to every organ in the body. This arrangement is simultaneously beneficial for diagnostic and therapeutic treatment of both body and soul. Through the manipulation of the areas left and right of the spinal cord, we can discover malfunctioning organs as well as the specific spiritual risk factors connected to the particular vertebrae.

With this wisdom we understand that for a complete holistic healing, it is not enough to treat diseases solely on a physical level. Holistic healing always requires a search for the spiritual risk factors that caused the disease and the help of the corresponding spiritual healing factors for the soul in order to overcome sickness of body and soul. Any attempt to suppress only the symptoms leads inevitably to an armada of sicknesses and symptoms that are usually chronic and incurable.

Ignorance of spiritual wisdom is very expensive for patients and beneficial only to the medical community and for the profit of the pharmaceutical industry. This book can help us acquire the spiritual wisdom and understanding to become personally responsible for ourselves and our sicknesses, so that we stay well and in good spirits.

Virtues and Vices

This table summarizes the relationship between spiritual risk factors and their corresponding bodily ailments. The survey of physical disorders is a short selection of the many possible autoaggressive sicknesses. The symbols come directly out of the visions of Hildegard and represent symptoms.

Negative Forces (Vices)	Positive Forces (Virtues)	Vertebra	Organ/System Physical Disorder	Symbol
1. Material Love	Heavenly Love	C1	Eyes Inflammation, infection, arthritis	Fire, embers, worms, snakes
2. Petulance	Discipline	C2	Ears, liver Infection, asthma	Fire, worms, smog
3. Love of Entertainment	Love of Simplicity	C3	Nose, larynx, trachea Asthma, hay fever, colds	Fire, smoke, smog
4. Hard-heartedness	Compassion	C4	Mouth, bronchi, lungs, heart Arteriosclerosis	Dry fountain, boiling tar, smoke, worms, red-hot nails
5. Cowardice	God's Victory	C5	Skin Herpes, psoriasis, shivers and fever	Black fog, rainstorms, fireballs
6. Anger	Tranquillity	C6	Immune system Autoaggression, viral infection	Fire, windy storm, black sea, mud, decay, worms
7. Inappropriate Mirth	Yearning for God	C7	Lymphatic system Back pain, viral infection	Swamp, bad-smelling smoke, fog, worms
8. Gluttony	Abstinence	Th1	Stomach and intestinal system, heart	Fire, ocean, sulfur Leaky-gut syndrome
9. Bitterness of Heart	Generosity	Th2	Intestinal system, gallbladder, heart Inflammation, allergies	Infernal fire, snakes

Negative Forces (Vices)	Positive Forces (Virtues)	Vertebra	Organ/System Physical Disorder	Symbol
10. Wickedness	Devotion	Th3	Stomach and intestinal system Gastro-cardiac symptoms, gas, constipation, bleeding hemorrhoids	Fire, red-hot lead, embers, fire-spitting dragon
11. Lying	Truth	Th4	Stomach and intestinal system Gastro-cardiac symptoms, ulcers, cancer, polyps	Black fire, embers, dragon, ice-cold water
12. Contention	Peace	Th5	Stomach and intestinal system, liver, bile ducts, pancreas Colitis, gastritis, Crohn's disease	Swamp, fog, hot storm, worms
13. Unhappiness	Blessedness	Th6	Stomach and intestinal system, pancreas Colitis, gas, cancer	Sulfuric fire, deep pits, worms
14. Immoderation	Discretion	Th7	Stomach and intestinal system, liver, biliary tract, pancreas Heartburn, gastritis, colitis	Burning fire, sulfur, gigantic ocean
15. Doom	Salvation	Th8	Stomach and intestinal system, liver, biliary tract, pancreas Migraine, asthma, pre-cancer, fibromyalgia, sciatica	Satanic abyss
16. Arrogance	Humility	Th9	Small and large intestines, liver, pancreas, muscles, nerves, joints Inflammation, infection	Fire, embers, big worms

Negative Forces (Vices)	Positive Forces (Virtues)	Vertebra	Organ/System Physical Disorder	Symbol
17. Envy	Charity	Th10	Kidneys, suprarenal glands, intestines, liver Immune deficiency, autoaggression, cancer, AIDS, multiple sclerosis, polyarthritis	Burning volcano spitting fire and lava, vipers, shivers, cold, fog, scorpions
18. Thirst for Glory	Reverence for God	Th11	Stomach and intestinal system Kidney disorders, inflammation, gas	Swamp, filth, worms, stink
19. Disobedience	Obedience	Th12	Intestines, back, legs, feet, kidneys Phlebitis, leg ulcers	Gloomy darkness, burning floor, biting worms
20. Lack of Faith	Faith	L1	Back, intestines, kidneys, ovaries, vagina, testes, penis, prostate, urinary tract, bladder Sciatica, stomach and intestinal disorders, depression, insomnia	Fire, darkness, stinking shit, worms
21. Desperation	Hope	L2	Back, intestines, uterus, testes, penis, prostate, urinary tract, bladder Back pain, gallbladder infection, appendicitis	Fire, pit, stink
22. Obscenity	Chastity	L3	Back, intestines, uterus, testes, penis, prostate Rheumatism, sexual disorders, insomnia, gas, autoaggression	Fire, glowing embers, sulfur, stink, decay, worms

Negative Forces (Vices)	Positive Forces (Virtues)	Vertebra	Organ/System Physical Disorder	Symbol
23. Injustice	Justice	L4	Back, intestines, uterus, ovaries, vagina, testes, penis, prostate Rheumatism, sciatica, osteomyelitis, back pain	Barbs and thorns, worms, burning rods
24. Lethargy	Fortitude	L5	Back, intestines Back pain, asthma, depression, nerve pain	Fire, dark layer of air, burning rods, demons
25. Oblivion	Holiness	S1	Back, rectum Back pain, lumbago, sciatica, colitis, phlebitis, colon cancer	Enormous fire, deep valley, stink, worms
26. Instability	Stability	S2	Back, urinary tract, bladder Weakness of the immune system, urinary infection, autoaggression	Fire, dragon
27. Concern for Worldly Goods	Heavenly Desire	S3	Back, sex organs Back pain, rheumatism, inflammation, infection	Fire, black flames, worms
28. Obstinacy	Remorse	S4	Back, external genitals Arteriosclerosis, cerebral sclerosis, stroke, heart attack, Alzheimer's disease	Darkness, tar, sulfur, cries of pain
29. Craving	Letting Go	S5	Back, genitals Back pain, cystitis, dropsy, kidney disease, obsession, addiction	Fire, embers, deep and gigantic ocean, dragon, demons

Negative Forces (Vices)	Positive Forces (Virtues)	Vertebra	Organ/System Physical Disorder	Symbol
30. Discord	Concord	Coccyx 1	Back, genitals Back pain, umbago, sciatica, rheumatism, mental disorder	Fire, fog banks, worms, demons
31. Scurrility	Reverence	Coccyx 2	Lower back, genitals Spinal disorders, immune deficiency, autoaggression	Fire, flames, worms
32. Vagabondage	Stability	Coccyx 3	Lower back, genitals Colitis, colon cancer, gas	Swamp, stink and decay, putrefying garbage, smelly fog
33. Occultism	Dedication to God	Coccyx 4	Genitals Sexual disorders, metabolic disorders, hormone disturbances	Fire, gigantic swamp, stink, snakes, worms
34. Avarice	Satisfaction	Coccyx 5	Lower back, genitals Metabolic disturbances, diabetes, thrombosis, embolism, depression, Weak nerves	Burning layer of air, embers, worms, wind, demons
35. Melancholy	Heavenly Joy	Skull	Head, heart Mental disorders, angina pectoris, depression, suicide	Desert, worms, darkness, burning rods

Turning the Evil into the Virtuous

Sometimes severe pain and hard work are necessary for spiritual growth from the dark side of our thirty-five egotistic weaknesses into the greater, more powerful side of the divine nature. Cultures worldwide use initiation ceremonies to train their youth in the value system of their tradition. The Aborigines in central Australia, for example, used controlled pain during initiation ceremonies to prepare their youth for extreme conditions in order to survive the relentless desert. Our Western multicultural society has only a few mutual values—that is, values that are important for everybody. Our world is already so dark from materialistic selfishness that it needs stronger measures like sickness, disaster, pain, and suffering to change into a brighter spirit and to reconnect with the divine nature.

The transition from the limited dark side into the greater values of inner richness requires us to overcome obstacles and suffering. Suffering and the dark side of our existence can teach us spiritual values such as love, discipline, compassion, and patience in order to force us into a greater spiritual realm. According to the law of opposites, we need sickness and weakness so they can be transformed into health and strength. The intensive experience of the negative side can sometimes establish its opposite. The ego experiencing death learns to give birth to life. To establish real spiritual life we have to let go of the old selfish nature. According to John 12:24, "Unless a kernel of wheat falls to the ground and dies, it remains only a single seed. But if it dies, it produces many seeds." In Goethe's words, "Stirb und werde!" (Die and come alive!)

Hildegard describes the consequences of a negative spiritual life by using visionary symbols for the resulting sicknesses. Each spiritual weakness and vice has its typical symbolic pattern.

- Fire is a tool to burn sickness into health, just as fever burns bacteria and viruses during an infection.
- Worms are used through decay and putrefaction to turn negative risk factors into virtuous values. Disease strengthens the immune system by burning enemies and intruders.

- Sulfur and stink are symbols for gas and malnutrition transformed by better diet and intestinal cleansing.
- Darkness and smog or fog are negative symbols to describe breathlessness, autoaggression, suffering, and death changed through intestinal cleansing, liver regeneration, and better nutrition to promote rebirth and a spiritual new beginning.
- The dragon is the personification of our own habits, addictions, and obsessions that put us voluntarily in our own prison. The slaying of the dragon by angelic forces rescues the captive soul from its addiction and frees the spiritual personality from obsession.
- The snake symbolizes renewal during the sloughing away of its skin. The new skin shows clearly the renewing and healing process after severe skin disorders such as neurodermitis, psoriasis, and acne, all of which are autoaggressive in origin.

In this respect the thirty-five vices and their related sicknesses are our teachers, instructing us to become more aware of our spiritual nature. Difficulties and suffering are inevitable in every life. But they are possibilities and opportunities to provide our limited egoistic selves a greater relationship with our real natures. Many people, including such creative geniuses as Beethoven, van Gogh, and Schubert, have reached the highest point of creativity and spirituality by going through tremendous suffering. Like them, we too should always look for the secret message in every evil and turn sickness into health, weakness into strength, and an enemy into a friend.

The Healing Power of Precious Stones and Crystals

Today there is a new technology for healing based on the application of the electric-magnetic energy transmitted by crystals and precious stones. The crystalline structure not only is an oscillator providing precise and regular frequencies but also has the capacity for tremendous information storage with endless possibilities.

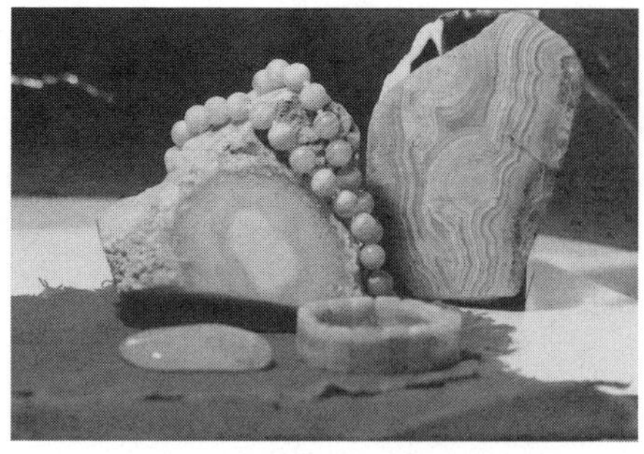

Crystals have changed the world in their use in the development of computer technology and of radio and television technique; for laser application in technology and surgery; for solar energy systems; and for transmitting large quantities of information over long distances via fiber-optic cables. Silicon cells are found in everything that stores unlimited information disseminated through the cosmic internet. Crystals carry specific information, just as does a floppy disk for a computer program.

There are many reports of ancient civilizations using crystals for healing or producing energy. Throughout history, crystals and gemstones were used as authoritative objects for religions and religious leaders to control human life.

THE PRESENCE OF THE TRINITY

Hildegard describes the presence of life energy in crystals and precious stones from the first day of Creation. Lucid creative energy entered the crystals in the form of the oscillation of tiny atoms on the crystalline structure, symbolizing the power of God the Creator. In the same way, every crystal is the visible form of the invisible God representing the power of Jesus Christ. The Holy Spirit is the third power existing in every precious stone, as seen by its beauty, spellbinding nature, and healing power.

The same cosmic energy is present in all matter of creation and contains the Creator's light and energy. Each cell on earth and each planet in the universe oscillates with the same vibrational energy as the precious stones. With this vibrational energy, the weak can be strengthened and deficient body cells filled with new life energy to maintain health and heal sicknesses.

HEALING WITH CRYSTALS AND PRECIOUS STONES

The crystal therapy of Hildegard of Bingen is an effective energetic medicine to bring body and soul into equilibrium. Crystal bioenergy can remove suffering and pain from nerves, muscles, and bones as it balances and cleanses the body and its organs. The healing energy in precious stones and crystals absorbs the negative energy of abnormal thoughts, emotions, and spiritual weaknesses and then transfers only positive natural bio-crystalline energy. Many stress-related illnesses stem from a negative and disharmonious thought system and a spiritual blackout.

Quartz crystals are capable of collecting sun energy and focusing the energy over the solar plexus to regenerate and empower the autonomic nervous system. Crystal water prepared with a sun-activated rock crystal is an effective cleansing and healing elixir for the thyroid gland and regulates hormones associated with that gland.

Other crystals, like the amethyst, transmit their healing power over the skin to control hematoma and coagulation as well as spiritual and emotional processes.

Crystal therapy can be helpful against anxiety, depression, distress, and other mental disorders. The neurological influence of crystals and their tranquilizing effect on the brain can be observed in the electroencephalogram (EEG), which has been recorded under the influence of the Gold Topaz Prayer (see page 224).

The emerald represents the entire vital energy, called *viriditas,* the power of the color green. The emerald helps to repair damaged cellular structures and supports wound healing on the molecular level, such as with chronic leg ulcers and other slow-healing wounds.

All precious stones and crystals carry healing energy that can be transformed not only to every cell of our bodies but also, and more important, to the weak energy system of our soul. Because diseases have a mostly spiritual origin, precious stones provide us with the tremendous healing power needed to repair the defect energy pattern of the soul.

Chapter 1

Principles of Hildegard's Psychotherapy

The Cosmic and Divine Forces of the Human Soul

1. Vision: The Cosmic Dimension of Humanity (LDO, Vision 3)

Four hundred years before the English physician and anatomist William Harvey (1578–1657) discovered that blood circulates throughout the body, Hildegard of Bingen described in a vision the circulation of the humors.

THE FOUR ELEMENTS AND THE FOUR HUMORS

> Thereupon, I saw how the humors in the human organism are distributed and altered by various qualities of the wind and the air, because the humors take on the same qualities. (LDO, Vision 3:1)

Hildegard's medicine is *humoral pathology*. Our health is a result of the quality of the humors, a metaphor for good humor and well-being. Especially in her medical textbook *Causae et Curae,* Hildegard describes body fluids such as blood, hormones, and semen and the metabolism of organs, which she calls *phlegma et livores:* "There are four humors. Two are the more predominant phlegms; the other two are biles" (CC 50:31).

"Mankind is peaceful and enjoys excellent physical health when the four humors are well balanced and in the right order. . . . The four humors in balance are like the four elements of the world" (CC 56:34).

The four humors have been well known in the field of medicine for many centuries. They are mentioned by physicians from Hippocrates to Paracelsus, but are described differently by Hildegard. For Hildegard, the four humors are the key to understanding the art of healing. The number four is significant not only in construction of the cosmos and the four world elements, but also in the makeup and function of human beings—for example, in the four temperaments and their characteristic variations in man and woman, as well as in the four blood types. The four humors are responsible for either illness or good health.

Like the animals of the four centers of direction, the humors change their conditions:

> The humors behave just like a leopard that sometimes roars wildly within us and other times is quiet. Such humors crawl forward or backward like a crab, thus signifying our changeability. They can behave like a stag, whose leaping thrusts are a sign of contradiction. At other times they have the predatory nature of a wolf. . . . They may behave like a lion to show their unconquerable power or may resemble a serpent, which can be either gentle or angry. They may also pretend to be mild as a lamb. Often they may growl within us like an angry bear. Thus the condition of humors is changed in many different ways. (Vision 3:1)

Hildegard sees further that the organs communicate with the help of the humors—for example, liver and brain, liver and ear. This knowledge is in Hildegard's medicine very important, both for natural diagnoses and for therapy:

> The humors often reach the human liver, where our perception, which comes from the brain, is tested. . . . If the blood vessels of the liver are affected by humors, they will disturb the vessels of the ear and can cause hearing disturbances, because good health or disease is often connected to our hearing ability. (Vision 3:1)

Hildegard sees the function of the autonomic nervous system and the solar plexus as a steering center for the organs:

> I also saw how the humors eventually reached the navel. The navel is the center of our intestines and keeps them under control. It provides body temperature and regulates the movements of our intestines, without which we could not live. (Vision 3:1)

Bodily fluids and hormones stimulate our sex organs and provide pleasure in sexual activity. There are no taboos for Hildegard, even though she lived in chastity, because sex is a gift of God.

> The humors also reach the sex organs, which can sometimes become playful or dangerous. . . . They are under the control of common sense, so you don't know what to do or what not to do. In this way we take pleasure in sexual activity. (Vision 3:1)

How can Hildegard know the function of the kidneys, the portal veins, the renal arteries, or vessels like the saphenous veins without having studied anatomy? All this is proof of her visionary gifts:

> The vessels of the brain, heart, lungs, and liver as well as those of the other organs give our kidneys strength, while the vessels of the kidneys descend to the calves of the legs and give them power. If the humors then ascend through the vessels of the legs, they unite with the male or female sex organs and provide them with potency. (Vision 3:1)

Sicknesses like headaches and epilepsy may occur when the humors dry out:

> If the humors are disturbed in an unnatural way and then affect the liver such that their moisture is lessened and lung humidity is diminished, illnesses occur. If our phlegm also turns dry and poisonous and rises to the brain, headaches or eye disturbances can occur. When in addition bone marrow dries out and the moon is on the wane, epilepsy can affect us. Our flesh becomes ulcerous as if we have leprosy [psoriasis] when the moisture around the navel dries out. . . .

At times the humors flow excessively through the chest and as a result flood the liver [with black bile], which can cause melancholy and madness. If these melancholic humors ascend to the brain, they may attack it [causing a stroke]. . . . If they descend to the stomach, they cause fever [and gastritis]. . . .

People can be sick for a long time. . . These humors can press against the small vessels of the ear [causing tinnitus] . . . with excessive phlegm they can attack the lung, and with the same mucus induce an attack of coughing such that one is scarcely able to breathe [asthma]. When the same humors extend to the vessels of the heart, they can cause heart pain [angina pectoris]; they can also spread to the side regions and cause inflammation of the lung [pleurisy].

The humors can flood around the navel, whereas the viscera like liver, pancreas, and intestines ascend to the brain and cause madness. An aggressive depression may occur if the humors also affect the gallbladder and increase the acidity of the blood through gallic acid.

Sometimes the humors, with their unsuitable moisture, overflow into the vessels of the kidneys and the calves of the legs and other parts of the body. If someone on top of that eats and drinks too much, the humors will destroy the muscles and cause swelling and pain [fibromyalgia, rheumatism, and gout]. Someone with balanced humors, not too moist and easily flowing through all the parts of the body, will stay healthy and grow in perception for good or for evil. (Vision 3:1)

THE ORIGIN OF AUTOAGGRESSIVE DISEASES

Eighty percent of the population of the Western world suffers and dies from illnesses such as cardiovascular disease, cancer, arthritis, hepatitis, and colitis, which are all classified as autoaggressive. There is virtually no organ or tissue in the human body that cannot be destroyed by aggression through our own immune system. But what makes us autoaggressive? Why do we commit suicide in a world of overabundance and material wealth?

Hildegard says it is the lack of spiritual power and absence of cosmic life energy, which she calls *viriditas,* the power of greenness. We become weak and unjust and live in oblivion and ignorance of God and of creation. The autoaggression reflects the sadomasochistic mentality in our global-player society: death and ethnic cleansing instead of living together in peace and harmony. All foundations on earth and in the universe are shaken by our Western society, and we become autoaggressive.

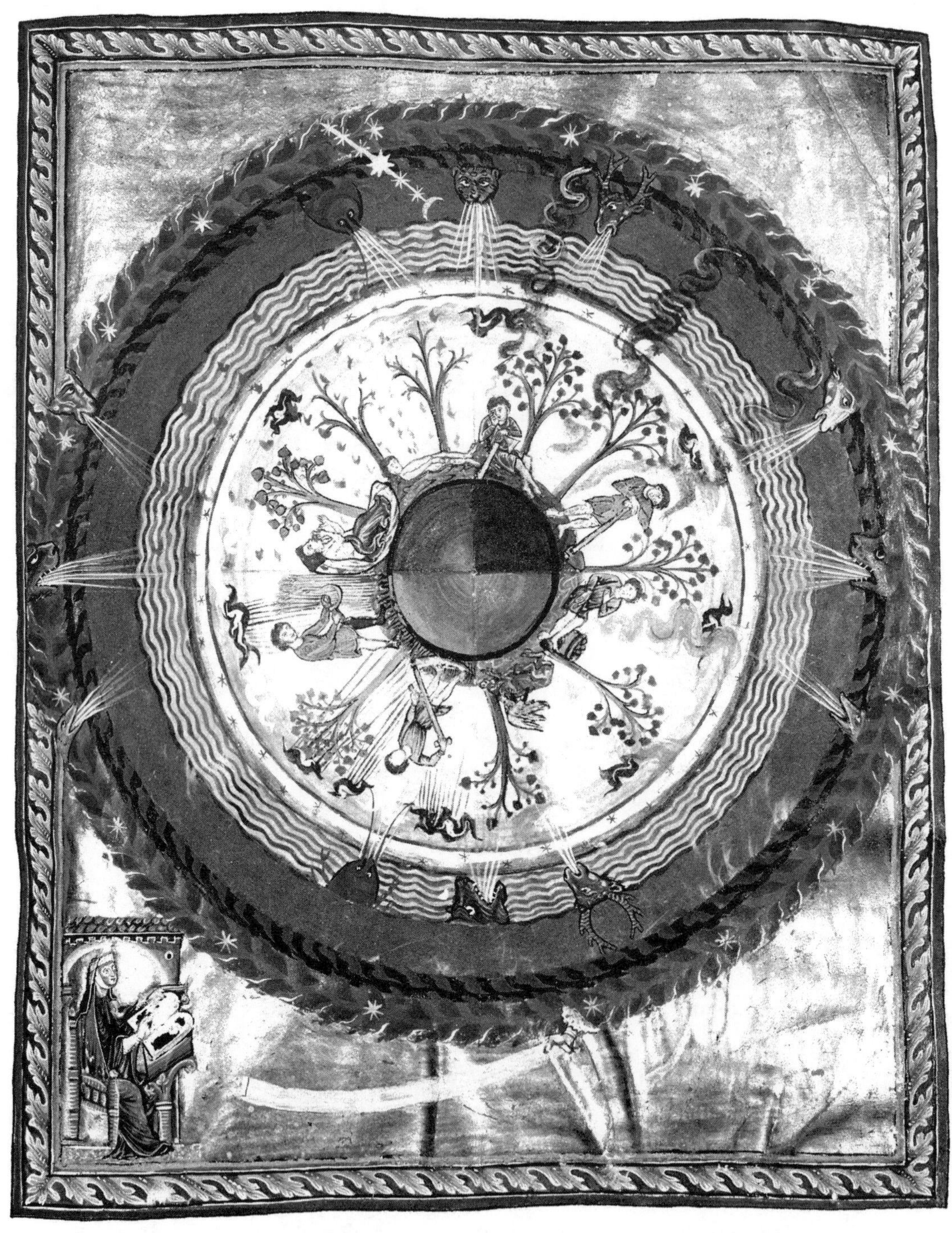

The Cosmic Apotheosis. There is no final death in the universe; every death is a circular transition to a new life. (LDO, Vision 4)

> Because our thoughts grow desolate, we go astray. Then the humors in the human organism become unnaturally excited and affect the liver [with production of gallic acid]. When the moisture of the vessels in the breast decrease and humors dry out, people get sick and as a result the muscles become ulcerous. Such people look like lepers. If the vessels of the sex organs are overstimulated, the proper moisture of the entire organism dries up. Pustules develop and we abandon the Holy Spirit as our sins fester in evil habits. The vitality of honorable deeds dries up within us and bad deeds will be exalted in a foul manner. (Vision 3:15)

The cosmic elements, heat and flooding, hurricanes and earthquakes will punish us until we return to love and cosmic responsibility. Only then, finally, will humanity recover and become healthy. Only then will the dew of the Holy Spirit sprinkle us with the dew of justice and virtuous power, because the universe works by laws of justice and harmony. At that time we will become brothers and sisters of God.

> If our thoughts are neither too reckless, nor too superficial, nor stubborn but rather harmonize well in the sight of humanity and God in honorable morality, then these thoughts will cause us to assume peaceful habits and be well grounded in wisdom. We will not care anymore for the applause of the world but instead, with the help of the virtues, sigh for heavenly joy, as it is written in the Song of Songs 7:12: "How beautiful are your feet in their sandals, O prince's daughter!"
>
> In other words, O you who rejoice in your heart and long for God in the good deeds through which you have hope of eternal life, your joy glows like the sunrise. You demonstrate to all other people a beautiful mode of life on the way to the Son of God. Then your soul is called a prince's daughter of the one who is called the Prince of Peace. (Vision 3:19)

You will see how cosmic you are because "God and humanity are united, like soul and body, because God created us in his image. The entire celestial harmony is a mirror of the harmony between God and humans, a mirror of all the miracles of God" (CC 65:22).

2. VISION: HUMANITY IN THE RHYTHM OF THE FOUR ELEMENTS

(LDO, VISION 4)

When God created humanity he used the same method by which he had created the universe. The microcosm represented by the human body is an exact miniature of the macrocosm, which is an image of the living power of the Creator itself.

THE COSMIC RELATIONSHIP OF HEALING AND SPIRITUALITY

> God formed humanity according to the divine image and likeness. He had in mind that this form should enclose the Holy Godhead. For the same reason, God included all of creation in the human form, just as the whole world emerged from the divine Word. (Vision 4:14)

What is the Word that carries creative energy? According to Hildegard and the authority of the Bible, this Word is the name of God, JHVH. The name of God is called the tetragrammaton, from the Greek *tetra* (four) and *gramma* (letter). There are four Hebrew letters used for the most powerful and sacred name of God. The tetragrammaton contains the blueprint from which the entire universe of matter and energy, time and space, humans and angels is made. The pronunciation of the name was sacred and secret, known only to the ancient Jewish high priests in Solomon's temple, and was lost after the fall to the Romans in A.D. 70.

The name has many meanings. The Jews were directed to speak the name Adonai (Lord) or Elochim, the Omnipotent, "He who is always the same" or "He who calls events into existence" but also "He who makes winds to blow."

THE NUMBER 4

In Hildegard's vision the number 4 corresponds perfectly with the name. Four! It is the number of the cosmic wheel and all creation:

- four elements, the building blocks of the universe
- four directions
- four seasons

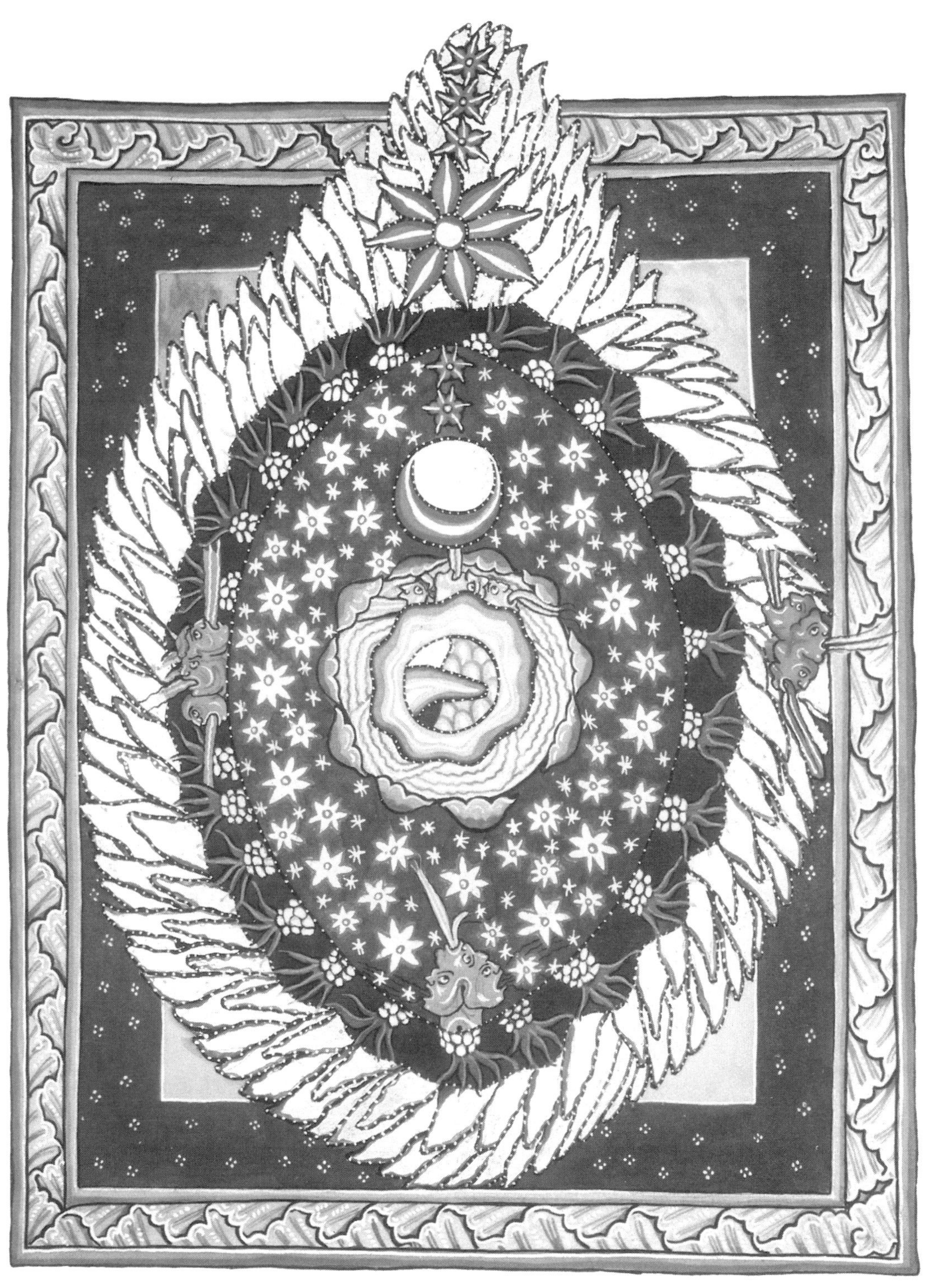

The Four Elements—Building Blocks of the Universe and of the Human Soul.

- four temperaments of humanity
- four humors of the human body
- four blood types—A, B, AB, and O
- four bases of the genetic code: adenine, cytosine, guanidine, and thymine, which together form 80,000 human genes
- the digital storage systems in computers and CDs

Four is also the visible number in two dimensions by the square and the cube. Four is 3, symbol for the Trinity, plus 1 for humanity. Four makes the three corners of the triangle unstable. This includes the possibility of humanity to live in harmony or destroy creation with its free will.

But God gave humanity all the creative potential to be his cocreator. Our growing awareness of nuclear and other ecological disasters is waking us up to refocus on Hildegard's visions about God the Creator and the return to life-sustaining wisdom in creation. Creation is an ongoing activity as long as life goes on. Creation is not a static event that happened long ago, once upon a time—it is continually evolving. According to Hildegard, creation is dynamic now and here, day after day, in our one body. Creation is our future and we are responsible cocreators with God, because we are made with the power of the divine in us.

Human beings are by nature creative. We are all responsible for building the city of God, the new Jerusalem, out of precious stones, with golden gates that are never closed. We ourselves are building blocks for that city of God.

HILDEGARD CELEBRATES HUMANITY

> God created the world out of its elements to the glory of the divine name. God strengthened it with the wind, connected it to the stars and enlightened it by them, and filled it with all manner of creatures. God then surrounded and fulfilled humankind in the world with all things and gave them tremendous power, so that all creation would support them in all things. Humankind cannot live without nature. (LDO, vision 4)

We are all cosmic by nature.

> God has formed humanity according to the pattern of the firmament

> and strengthened human power with the strength of the elements. God has the power of the universe firmly adapted to us so that we breathe, inhaling and exhaling these forces, like the sun, which illuminates the earth. . . . Thus the roundness and symmetry of the human head signifies that while the soul sins according to the desires of the flesh, it will then regenerate itself in repentance. . . . As long as body and soul live with each other, they will put up with conflicts. The soul suffers whenever the flesh rejoices in sinning. (Vision 4:16)

THE SOUL REMEMBERS IT CAME FROM GOD

> The soul is so deeply within us that it seems our body is animated of its very self. The soul knows it comes from the Creator and calls God by many names. (Vision 4:18)

The soul has two capacities: one to work and act, the so-called *sympaticus,* and one to recuperate and rest, called the *parasympaticus.* These two capacities correspond to the old Benedictine wisdom of *Ora et labora,* pray and work in balanced amounts.

> The soul has two capacities, to equalize and control stress and to release its passionate activity. Through contemplation, the soul ascends to the heights, where it experiences God. Through activity the soul works with the entire body to achieve its goals. The soul enjoys operating in the body because God has formed it, and this is why the soul is eager to fulfill the work of the body.
>
> The soul regulates the functions of the body; it ascends into the brain, the blood, and the bone marrow. The soul can operate only within the limits of the body, and it cannot accomplish more than divine grace permits. Often the soul works for the desire of the flesh until the sweat flows and the flesh dries up. At such a time the soul becomes inactive until it can be regenerated, warming up the blood and renewing the bone marrow. When the body pursues only its desires, often disgust will grow, but when the body is regenerated, it will also renew the soul to the service of God. (Vision 4:20)

Hildegard reveals the relationship of our nervous system to the planets. Billions of nerve cells are connected day and night with the power plant of the universe and receive tremendous amounts of life and regenerative energy. These nerve points are the seven chakras of Hildegard's medicine.

> From the top of our cranium to the forehead are found seven points, separated from one another by equal parts. They symbolize the seven planets, which are also separated from one another. The highest planet, the sun, has its spot on the top of the cranium. In the place between the eyebrows is the moon. Between sun and moon Mercury and Venus are located on the forehead, and Mars, Jupiter, and Saturn can be found on the back of the head. This signifies that from the very beginning the soul accomplishes its deeds with the seven gifts of the Holy Spirit, which are radiated to us by the seven planets. (Vision 4:22)

The energy of the seven planets is connected to our nervous system and shows the strong relationship between our soul and the universe.

> In this way the soul directs the body. The soul is a rational spirit. Its wisdom resides in the heart. The wisdom by which the soul thinks and acts is like the patriarch of a family taking care of its affairs. The soul has a fiery nature to heat up all the vital life processes in the body. (Vision 4:25)
>
> A human being has two natures; it is heavenly in its soul and earthly in its body. It is the perfect work of God and knows both earthly and heavenly things, and is aware of heaven through faith. (Vision 4:92)

The holistic approach to the human being needs to understand how body and soul work together.

> In this way God has strengthened us with all the power of nature. He gave us perceptive tools to recognize the world through our sight, understand through our hearing, and distinguish through our sense of smell. As a result we will be nourished by the world and master it by our sense of touch. We experience through our five senses the true God, who is the author of creation. Thus God has formed us according to the master plan of the universe, just like an artist who paints his models. And as God has made the giant instruments of the universe according to appropriate standards, divinity made humanity in equal but much shorter form. (Vision 4:97)

DIVINE LIFE ENERGY

We are always connected with the divine life energy, which flows through the universe. Lack of this life energy produces life-threatening consequences. The symptoms of disease are the visible signs of this lack in our body. Hildegard emphasizes that we are able to heal and regenerate with cosmic life energy via our soul. Each organ needs the cosmic bioenergy for its proper function. This message is the basis for a completely new cosmic therapy that we call cosmic *psychosynthesis*, in contrast to the usual psychoanalysis of today. The essence and the strength of Hildegard's medicine allows us to link up with all the spiritual energies of the universe.

> The soul contains a fiery substance (bio-photon-energy), which is why we are warm-blooded creatures. With this energy, the soul sustains the entire human organism and gives life to the body. The soul's path through the body is by nature a windy one. The soul inhales life energy and then exhales. We dry out by inhaling, which is good for us, as the flesh remains healthy and becomes revitalized as the result of the dryness. The fire of the body diminishes during exhalation; thus, warmth is removed. The entire body works with the greatest sensitivity to stay alive and makes use of all five senses. The fire of the soul would burn the body like a house in flames if the heat were not removed by breathing.
>
> The power of the soul surrounds the human body with flesh and blood to fulfill its function, just as the blowing of the winds ripens fruit on earth. We recognize God through the fiery quality of the soul and likewise our body functions through the breath of the spirit. In the same way, we received the law from God: to do rightly whatever we do.
>
> The soul is like the lady of the house. God has formed the human body so that the soul can live in it. No one can see the soul, just as we cannot see God, but faith enables us to become wise. The soul creates thoughts sent from God and produced in the heart. These thoughts are the written records of the soul, which ascend into the brain and from there into the entire body. The soul also enters the eyes, for the eyes are the windows to the soul and a bridge to the macrocosm.
>
> The soul nourishes the human organism and regenerates the entire body. The body flourishes by this supportive function and can maintain its good condition. The soul is not of flesh and blood itself, but it serves them and keeps them alive. The soul has its origin in God, who breathed

> life into the body. Body and soul exist, despite their differences, in one reality as a work of God. Humanity is a corporeal reality from the very beginning, from the top to the bottom, from the outside to the inside. Everywhere, in every respect, we exist in our one reality. (Vision 4:103)

Our destiny is eternity and the return to God our Father and Mother. This goal can be achieved only when we live in harmony with the universe.

> If we act responsibly, the elements will stay in balance, but if we fall into disrepair, the elements will suffer and react mightily. Body and soul work together in accordance with free will, but God judges us according to the results of our work.
>
> The soul blows like a draft in a house, spreading the power of thought, speech, and breath. The soul is tuned to earth as long as body and soul work together. The body cannot free itself from its ties to earth.
>
> On the day of judgment, the body will be renewed by its living soul and the body will become so light that it can fly. The soul is aware of God as long as it is associated with the body, even though it cannot see the invisible God. When the soul leaves the body and returns to God, it will recognize its own nature. At that point the soul will see the magnificence of its own dignity and require its body back so that the body, too, can enjoy its grandeur.
>
> When body and soul are reunited, they will appreciate God's glory in perfection. The angels will sing from this event in hymns of praise, just as they did on the first day of creation. . . . The hymns will proclaim the miracles bestowed by God on humanity. They will never cease to play upon the zither, in praies of the wonder God accomplished in humanity. This is the purpose of human nature. Humanity is one unit with soul and body, and it exists as the work of God in harmony with all of creation. (Vision 4:104)

3. Vision: Relationship between Body and Soul (SC, Vision 4)

Every one of us is a child of God. Our life begins when the soul, represented by a golden kite, enters the body in the mother's womb. Heaven and earth, the invisible and the visible, come together and a new human being is born.

Our divine soul looks like a golden kite that descends from a blue sky. Both gold and blue signify the royal power of God. The entire universe vibrates in gold and blue to show the presence of God's energy in his creation. "No creature, whether visible or invisible, lacks this royal life energy," writes Hildegard.

In this colorful illumination the golden kite has four corners, which represent the four directions and the four cosmic elements: fire, air, water, and earth. We burn with the cosmic fire to sustain our vital life energy, breathe the air to provide oxygen for the burning process of our metabolism, drink water for the humors and the body juices, and use earth to build bones and ligaments out of forty-five different minerals.

If we look closer, the four-cornered kite is divided into three parts symbolizing the three divine personalities of God, Christ, and the Holy Spirit. Together, four and three are the seven divine, cosmic forces that are the essence of our life center, the power that keeps us going and the center of our well-being. As long as we stay in tune with this energy, we are in harmony with God, the universe, and nature.

Life begins when this golden kite enters the body. That is when the infant starts moving. Hildegard describes the unification of body and soul as taking place approximately in the third month, when the mother feels the movements of her baby for the first time. From now on we are perfectly programmed, as Hildegard points out: "Naturram homine bonum est"—from nature woman and man are perfectly made.

FIREBALLS: SYMBOLS OF LIFE ENERGY

Hildegard's concept of fireballs as a symbol of life energy reveals the deepest secrets of creation. The same light energy that started creation on the first day is equivalent to the radiance of God, who brings the macro- and microcosmos into being. Hildegard calls this energy *lucida materia,* lucid energy that penetrates the physical matter—*turbulenta materia.* The transmission of the divine life energy throughout the universe carries information to all creatures over all time and space over long distances. Normal life is impossible without this divine energy, or radiation, that is present in human beings as well as in plants, animals, and minerals. According to

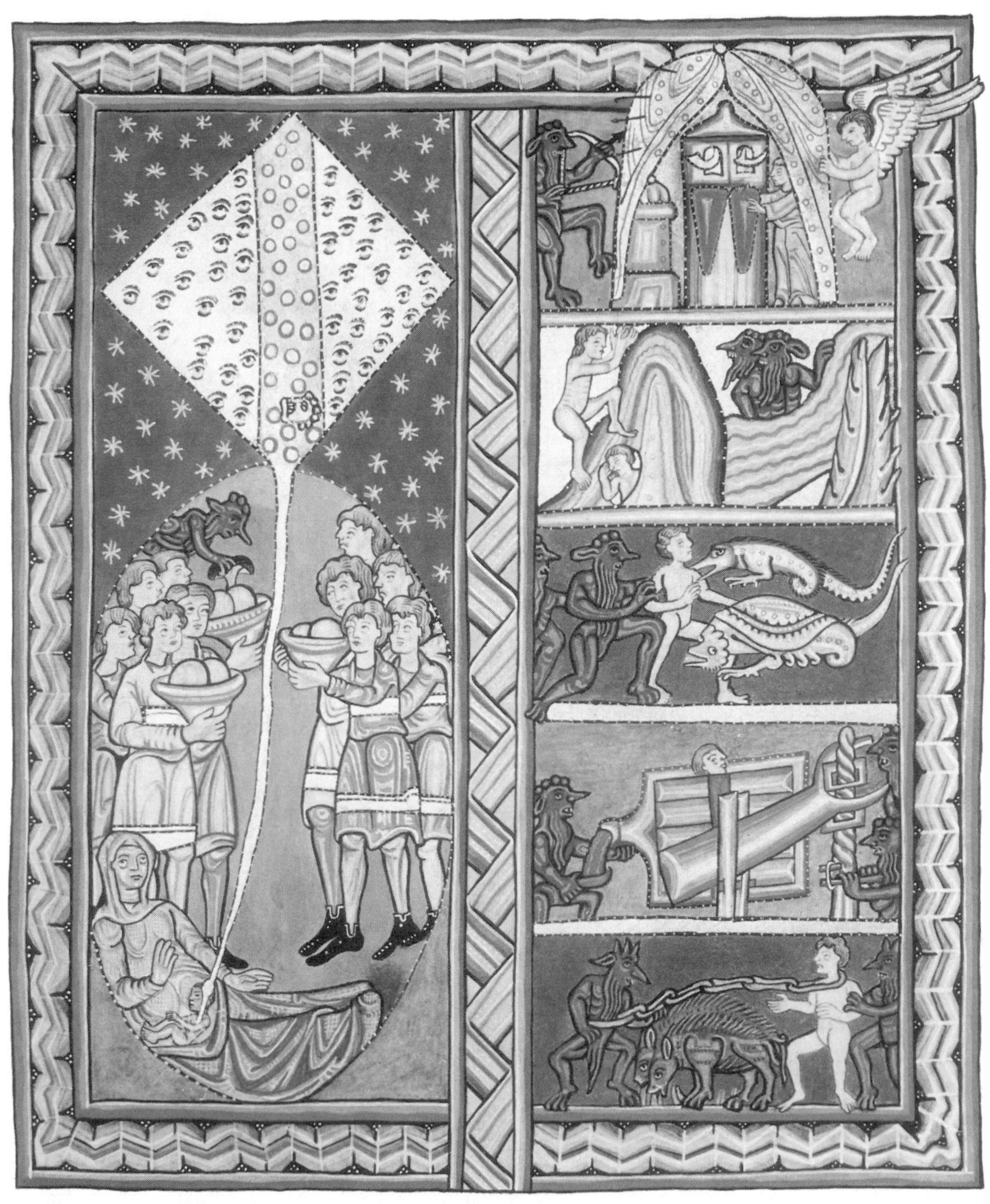

The Golden Kite of the Soul.

Hildegard, "No creature, whether visible or invisible, lacks this spiritual life energy."

The existence of a cosmophysical life force that rules macro- and microcosmic processes can be understood only since the biophysical discovery of light particles. The scientist and professor of quantum physics Fritz-Albert Popp, of the Institute of Biophysics in Germany, discovered the high-energy quanta and called it *biophoton,* a type of radiation that is absorbed by all living organisms. Studies show that all life processes are stimulated by biophotons, which penetrate the intercellular matrix of the DNA, our genetic code. The DNA of the cell regulates all life processes and relays thousands of bits of metabolic information with the help of this biophotonic language. The entire body speaks and understands it. This language—"the whispering of the stars and the whispering of the cells"—is characteristic of all processes in any nature of macro- and microorganisms.

THE MUSICAL LANGUAGE OF HARMONY: THE VOICE OF GOD

To understand the body's ability to function, let us examine a symphony orchestra. A harmonic sound is possible only when the conductor, the soloists, and all the different instrumentalists speak and understand the same language of music. Harmony is not possible if a single musician makes a mistake.

Divine energy operates in the same way: When all creatures speak and understand the language, information is transferred with 100 percent efficiency. The transfer of digital information bridges the gap between God and his creation. Hildegard's vision of fireball projectiles carrying the bioinformation to all living cells goes beyond the knowledge of her time—and also of today's dogmatic medicine. It opens a window for a new medicine and greater understanding of life in the future.

THE DIVINE CELL INFORMATION THERAPY

Every creature and the sun, moon, stars, plants, animals, and even minerals vibrate in the divine radiance and communicate with one another from distances of hundreds and thousands of miles. Disease is therefore a result of misinformation and a lack of biophotons. Negative feedback in living cells creates molecular chaos, which is responsible for the growth of malignant tumors, inflammatory diseases, and immune impairment like autoagression.

Healing occurs when the divine life energy reenters the impaired molecular DNA with the help of natural remedies that transmit biophotons. Herbs and plants, animals, and even precious stones are able to interact with our human cells via biophotons from their biosphere. Spiritual healing occurs when you lift your hands and ask God for help, pray, meditate, or go to a place with strong natural radiation. All these methods are the secret of healing success with Hildegard's medicine, which is based on proper nutrition, natural healing remedies, and constant communication with God. The biocommunication with biophoton signals to all living creatures provides a scientific basis for Hildegard's medicine and for healthcare in the future.

OUR MOTHER—TRANSMITTER OF SPIRITUAL LIFE

Only a woman is capable of receiving and giving life. This is Hildegard's greatest appreciation for her sisters and for the uniqueness of women. She writes: "Men are full of strong courage and strength; women are gifted with sensible spiritual strength." We understand through her vision that our birthplace is the earth, an intimate egg-shaped microcosmos integrated into the blue macrocosmos of the divine. The power of God enters his home, a little baby, through a golden navel string, a vision of inexplicable significance. Heaven and earth, body and soul, man and woman, God and humanity are united in every human being. We are all a center of divinity, a temple for God, who lives deep inside us.

Every newborn baby receives this gift of the royal personhood. The soul regulates all growth regulation and activities with this royal information. "The soul," writes Hildegard, "is in the body just as humors are in the tree, truly like the power of the tree bursting forth with its fruits." All the universe is an electromagnetic continuum of live energy that lives in the helix structure of DNA and regulates the entire organism. Day and night we are constantly connected with this energy system that keeps the whole body alive. We are more than just bone and flesh, cells and tissues; we live from the divine energy within us.

ILLUMINATION: BODY AND SOUL

In Hildegard's vision we see a pregnant woman. Three groups of men stand around her holding bowls with round balls of cheese, which represent the male semen. The men on the right-hand side carry strong semen like hard Swiss cheese. Their children will be strong and healthy with "great spiritual and fleshly gifts."

Each child is endowed with a wealth of spiritual and physical gifts from grandfathers and ancestors. They master their lives with prudence and discretion and benefit humanity. They are not prone to demonic forces.

The men on the left side are holding semen made of weak and soft cheese; their children will be weak and melancholic. There is a third kind of children who are made of bitter cheese that has been spoiled by a little devil mixing his poison in the male semen. These children will grow up to be malformed or slow-witted. Although suffering from lots of anguish and heart trouble, they can still grow up to be wonderful people. With the help of God these people will be crowned with victory, because God takes them personally under his guidance in the school of life and shows them the way to salvation, according to his word:

> I kill and I make alive; I wound and I heal;
> And there is none that can be delivered out of my hand.
>
> —Deuteronomy 32:39

All three kinds of children receive a divine soul, which is able to repair the genetic deformity responsible for inherited genetic disease. On the other hand, a normal genetic code is not necessarily a guarantee of health and well-being. Specialists in genetic medicine are in great error to believe that manipulated gene repair is necessary to rid the body of disease. The theory "one gene, one disease" ignores the fact that all cells participate in the divine biophoton transfer, which is greater than any manipulation of the genetic code practiced by genetic medicine of today.

SICK BUT ALWAYS HEALTHY

As important as genes and the genetic code are, vastly more important is the soul itself. Every one of us is endowed with a divine center, and this cosmic center is always complete and healthy and holy by nature, no matter how sick the body. This message is at the core of Hildegard's medicine!

Just as Hildegard predicted eight hundred years ago, genetic microbiology has discovered today that the single cell contains in its nucleus all the genetic information needed to create an entire new body. All characteristic human qualities of the body are stored in the blueprint of DNA, in more than 100,000 genes—a tremendous library of individual bits of information. The genetic material contains a master copy for the final new human being. Recent biophysics research shows how Hildegard's life energy concept can explain the way the cellular DNA matrix regulates all appropriate organs and builds the different nerve, bone and tissue cells by speaking the language of the divine, which today we call optical radiation via biophotons.

THE THREE FORCES OF THE SOUL

Will, intelligence, and emotion form the triad of the soul.

> A person has three essentials: the soul, the body, and the five senses. These make a person strong. The soul keeps the body alive and it breathes forth the senses. . . . You have eyes for seeing, ears for hearing, a heart for reflecting, hands for working, and feet for walking. Therefore, the senses are like precious stones. . . . The senses truly touch the soul, so the soul provides life to the body, just as fire lights the darkness.
>
> The soul can discern whether the work of people is good or evil. . . . The soul is an investigator. It inquires whether things are useful or useless, lovable or hateful, related to life or to death. . . .
>
> Similarly, the will is another power in the soul. The will is active and performs each action, whether it is good or evil. It is like a fire, cooking each meal as if it were in a furnace. The will can be likened to a baker who bakes bread to perfection.
>
> Actually, the soul with its will makes food better for people than bread. . . . While the soul remains in the body, the two work together either for good or for evil. . . . The soul rules the entire body by keeping it alive. . . . When someone does something evil, it is as bitter to the soul as poison is to the body. On the other hand, the soul rejoices in good, just as the body enjoys good food. The soul flows through the body as sap through the tree. Moisture keeps the tree green and produces flowers and fruits. That's why the soul is like sap in the tree. The green leaves symbolize

> understanding, the flowers the will, and the fruits burst forth as from the tree of intelligence. . . .
>
> The soul, whose essence is life, lives as a living fire in the body . . . . Thus, three basic powers exist with equilibrium in the soul: spirituality, knowledge, and sensibility to fulfill its functions. . . . These powers work in harmony, as none of them exceeds another. (Vision 4:17)

THE DARK SIDE OF LIFE

Life is not always joy and happiness; on the contrary, for the sake of joy and happiness there must be struggle, pain, and injury. Health does not hurt and is taken for granted, but everybody is thankful and happy when wounds are healing and the fight is over.

Life is not an easy way. The soul wanders and struggles, homeless, like a stranger in the shadow of death. Each of us goes through ups and downs, hills and valleys; stormy waves splash us back and forth, but God is always with us.

Hildegard is realistic about our daily life, which sometimes is not at all like a rose garden but more like a pigpen. We see under the golden tent four pictures that demonstrate what she means.

Man is a stranger in the shadow of death and walks the way of error. He is removed from the golden tent and led into a place of horror and cruelty. Chains bind him and he is thrown into the pigpen. He escapes but his enemies come again and put him into a winepress, where he is tortured and the last drop of blood is squeezed out. Again he frees himself but now more plagues appear in the form of scorpions, adders, and poisonous snakes, symbols of viral infections and other sicknesses. Hildegard describes the journey of the soul in despair:

"How can I break these chains? Who can free me from this prison? Whose eyes can look upon my wounds? Who has mercy for my pain? I am a stranger without any consolation and with no one to help me. Who will help me unless it is God? Where will I flee? My sorrow is immeasurable. I think about my wounds and suffering and weep and weep so much that all my wounds are covered with my tears."

Finally the soul cries for her mother, the female side of God, who shows her a narrow way by which she can escape into a little cave, symbol of the mother's uterus or the return to paradise, home.

A very sweet odor, smooth as gold, touches her nose. Now she has enough strength to leave the cave, and goes along a narrow footpath. But the footpath is full of thorns and other hindrances. Nevertheless, she reaches the top of the mountain and there she sees other obstacles—a foaming sea and rivers to prevent her crossing to the other side. More adders, scorpions, dragons, and other serpents start coming and thousands of little devils with their tongues sticking out are screaming: "Let us stir up our skills and surround her so carefully that she will not be able to flee from us again."

In her greatest despair the soul shrieks, terrified, to her mother and asks again for help: "O mother, where are you?"

And God does not rest. This time the mother provides her strongest support and gives the soul wings—symbols of mobility—to fly over the highest mountains. "Hurry," she says, "because God has given you wings to fly that nobody can stop. Therefore, fly quickly over all those poisonous and deadly beasts."

Gold Topaz Prayer

In remembrance of your divine origin, take a gold topaz in your hand, hold it each morning on your heart, and pray:

"Deus qui super omnia et in omnibus magnificatus est,
in honore suo me non abiiciat,
sed in benedictione me
conservet, confirmet, et constituat."

God who is glorified over everything and in everything,
in great reverence cast me not away from thy presence,
but in your blessing sustain, strengthen, and become one with me.

OUR SPIRITUAL JOURNEY TO THE GOLDEN TENT

We see on the top right of Hildegard's vision a person in a protective golden tent warming his hands at the fireplace. The devil is shooting arrows against him to no avail as the guardian angel on the right protects him.

Every person seeks his home on earth, a temple of God, a center of protection, a golden tent. Because of our royal personhood we receive a golden tent decorated with the sun and the stars, a tent of angelic glory with a floor of golden topaz. Gold is the color of God, the sun provides us with life energy, stars signify universal wisdom, and the tent is a symbol for our journey as a wanderer on earth. The golden tent reminds us of God, who holds his hand over our entire lives.

4. VISION: THE TRINITY IN THE UNITY (SC II, VISION 2)

PICTURE TRINITY AND THE HOLY SPIRIT?

For hundreds of years the discussion about the Trinity was of paramount importance. To imagine just how important this question was, we need to go back to the fourth century, when the emperor Constantine made it a state issue. In the first great ecumenical council in 325 and in the later council in Constantinople, the Nicene Creed—a synopsis of the Christian faith—was adopted, binding generation to generation throughout Europe.

A far richer understanding of the nature of the divine comes from Hildegard of Bingen, who pictures the divine Trinity in a gold and silver energy field around a sapphire blue Christ, a human person stretching out his hands to heal. The Trinitarian life energy flashes like electromagnetic vibrational energy. The fire of the golden Holy Spirit binds everything together: one light, three people, one God.

When this energy combines with matter, life comes into being, a very old wisdom in the mythology of native beliefs and a very new concept in modern relativity physics. Two mutually exclusive properties, energy and matter, coexist in this illumination of Hildegard's. The silver light signifies God, the Creator of life; the blue person Christ represents the Word made flesh; and the reddish golden color signifies the Holy Spirit, who is without any dryness, death, or darkness.

According to Hildegard, the divine Trinity can also be understood through a precious stone, a flame, or a word: "Three strengths are in a stone—moist greenness, tangibility, and reddish fire." The moisture is the creative healing power from God, which penetrates the body and is of the same strength as the energy in our nervous system. Tangibility stands for the Word made palpable after birth. The reddish fire is the power of the Holy Spirit, who is the illuminator of our hearts, lighting up the darkness of ignorance.

Similarly, three powers are in a flame: the three aggregate states of solid, liquid, and gas symbolizing the Trinity. The candle consists of shining brightness, giving life as does God. The burning fire is the power of Christ, who creates healing wonders; the radiance is the power of the Holy Spirit spreading the fire of love. Finally, three forces are in a word: the thought, the sound, and the result. The thought is the word not yet spoken. The sound is the spoken word that can be heard. And the result is what happens after the word has been spoken. This fireball of the Trinity is also the holy dynamite bringing all creation into being.

COSMIC INFLUENCES

Hildegard foresees the collapse of the environment through pollution caused by satellites, airplanes, automobiles, and products from agribusiness and the pharmaceutical industry, as well as genetic engineering and genetic cloning. The price of scientific progress is very high—it can cost us our existence and the security of our homeland, the creation.

"We are now becoming aware how the winds are blowing toward the wheel and humanity . . . for the winds maintain the whole universe by their power, so that nothing breaks apart," writes Hildegard. "We will slowly begin to understand that all these things have a relationship to the salvation of our soul" (LDO 2:24).

Hildegard's prophetic visions inspire us to look for new energy sources to replace the environment-destroying ones of today. Wind power may be enough and could produce thirty-five times more energy than the whole of humankind needs. Together with solar and water energy, wind energy lasts forever. Demons block us from natural resources because we live in oblivion, forgetting completely creative spirituality and cosmic intelligence.

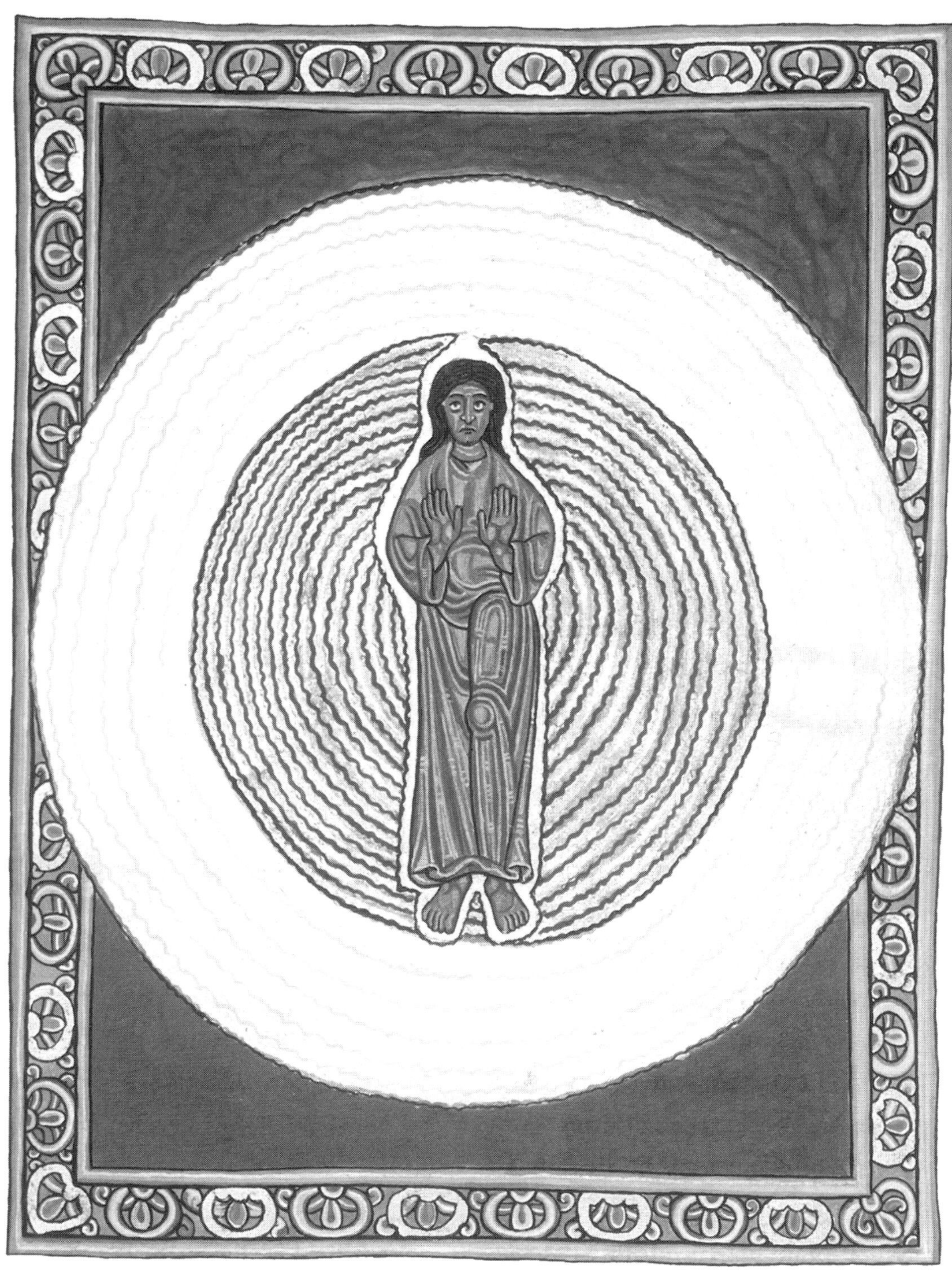

The Trinity in the Unity. The trinity is a gold and silver energy field around a sapphire blue Christ, all a symbol of our Spiritual life energy. (*Scivias II,* Vision 2)

TWELVE ANIMAL SPIRIT KEEPERS

From the four directions of the universe Hildegard sees the heads of twelve animals breathing onto the human figure: 2 crabs, a leopard, 2 stags, 2 lambs, 2 bears, a serpent, a wolf, and a lion. As they are in Native American beliefs, these animals are the spirit keepers standing for the "power of virtues" that keep humanity working in the universe and on earth: patient like a lamb, strong as a bear, clever like a serpent.

Hildegard writes: "The heads of the animals exhale forces of wind according to precise natural laws that spin the cosmic network throughout the world and create a corresponding moral relationship. All these animals breathe toward the wheel and these winds keep the universe in balance. . . . Neither the universe nor humanity could live without the blowing of the winds" (LDO 2:17).

Everybody who stays in tune with God and the universe receives an abundance of power. He who turns away lives in a spiritual blackout. Hildegard foresees our time as a period of forgetfulness. Western civilization is without this spiritual power because it lives oblivious to God and nature. This is the greatest disease of our time. It is responsible for our loss of meaning and also for violence and addiction to such things as work, alcohol, drugs, and sex that keep us occupied and make us neurotic. Nevertheless, all nonsense contains sense and every disease has the chance to be healed.

BEING INTERCONNECTED

Everything in the world teaches us that we are connected to God with body and soul, just as the seven planets—Mercury, Venus, the sun, the moon, Mars, Jupiter, and Saturn—have the task of influencing the power of the sun and moon.

"Each cosmic power is balanced by another one," writes Hildegard. "Thus every creature is linked to every other and each creature is in harmony with every other. In this respect the planets are auxiliary forces for the sun."

The influence of the moon also plays an important role:

"When the moon is waxing," Hildegard writes, "brain and blood of humans also increase. Correspondingly, they diminish when the moon wanes. We would fall into a terrible madness if the human brain always remained the same. If blood always had the same quality, we would also waste and die. When the moon is full, our brain is full and has the right potential. We are then in full possession of our senses. Under the new moon our brain is empty, without the full power of sensory forces. . . . And when the moon is in balance, we enjoy perfect health of brain and mind. The humors of the organism are balanced when the elements are in harmony, but they are out of balance, when the cosmic powers are disturbed, for humans could not exist without the balance and support of cosmic powers" (LDO 2:32).

We all receive our charismatic gifts from the power of the universe. Our billions of nerve cells are constantly connected with world intelligence:

"The seven planets signify the seven gifts of the Holy Spirit, which exceed all human reason" (LDO 2:33).

Our faith depends totally on our environment. Hildegard writes, "When the elements suffer under various catastrophes, then the light of the sun darkens like a solar eclipse. That is a sign and proof that our hearts and heads have turned to error. Then human beings are no longer walking the right path of nature but instead fight one another in many conflicts" (LDO 2:32).

Ecological and political crises are signs of separation from God the Creator. In contrast, a return to cosmic love is characterized by an inner sense of peace, security, and confidence that heals depression and anxiety. The love of the universe liberates us from today's worries, anger, madness, and neuroses and the collapse of our entire environment.

"Out of this real love," writes Hildegard, "which is totally divine, arises all goodness, which stands above everything else. Love attracts everybody who desires blessing" (LDO 2:46).

She continues, "Those who overcome shall be converted to goodness. Their wounds will be washed and the divine hosts will look down at the wounds that have been healed and will burst into songs of praise in honor of God. Realize that these words are proclaimed for the salvation of body and soul, not out of a human mouth, but by myself, the one 'I AM.'" (LDO 2:47).

Chapter 2

Spirituality and Healing

We are looking into the future to search for new values with quality standards that are applicable to the daily life of the third millennium. Our lives follow our own orientations, and the decisions we make are are arrived at according to our own values. But what are our values and who makes our decisions?

Ever since Adam and Eve ate from the tree of knowledge of good and evil, our lives have followed the same pattern of decision between two polarities or two possibilities. The principle of polarities is the basis of creation itself. We, too, decide through the principle of polarity and participate daily, like God, in the creation process.

Former generations were heavily influenced in their daily decisions by the values of their societies or of their families. Today, for the first time in history, there are only a few standards that are respected by everyone. Because we live in a multireligious and multicultural society, most people decide according to a narrow set of values or make no decision at all. Little mistakes can be corrected by life, but great mistakes tend to destroy life, relationships, health, or happiness. Our own lives are always a mirror of our own decision-making processes.

Is There a World Ethos?

Everyone, according to the science of the Creator *(Scientia Dei),* is a microcosm in the macrocosm and participates with the guidance of his soul in the process of the entire universe. The souls of all humans are a miniature of the macrocosm and a key to understanding the entirety. The soul receives the wisdom of the divine and contains a treasure of spiritual wealth.

Discovery of Cosmic Psychosomatic Values

In her first work, *Scivias* (Know the Way for Health and Healing), Hildegard explains the function and power principles of our souls. The soul contains the four cosmic life elements—fire, air, water, and earth—together with the three spiritual forces of the Trinity: God, the Son, and the Holy Spirit.

Hildegard wrote her psychotherapeutic book, *Liber Vitae Meritorum* (The Book of Life's Merits), when she was sixty years old, after her two medicinal books, *Causae et Curae* (The Causes and Therapies) and the *Physica,* a book on the healing forces in nature. *Liber Vitae Meritorum* reveals the conflict of the soul between thirty-five positive spiritual forces and thirty-five negative forces. She calls the decision making between those forces the struggle between virtues and vices. The virtues reflect the condition of the divine world; the vices represent the conflicts in our daily lives. Each weakness is counterbalanced by a positive strength as summarized in the table on page 40.

Practical Application of Hildegard's Psychotherapy

The application of the thirty-five virtues in our daily life enables us constantly to receive thirty-five health-promoting forces. The negative partners are psychosomatic risk factors and can cause physical disorders leading to chronic disease. No one can be cured without the correction of the defect in the appropriate area.

Liber Vitae Meritorum (The Book of Virtues and Vices)

	Vices	Virtues
1.	*Amor saeculi* (material love)	*Amor caelestis* (heavenly love)
2.	*Petulantia* (petulance)	*Disciplina* (discipline)
3.	*Joculatrix* (love of entertainment)	*Verecundia* (love of simplicity)
4.	*Obduratio* (hard-heartedness)	*Misericordia* (compassion)
5.	*Ignavia* (cowardice, resignation)	*Divina victoria* (God's victory)
6.	*Ira* (anger, criminality)	*Patientia* (tranquillity)
7.	*Inepta laetitia* (inappropriate mirth)	*Gemitus ad Deum* (yearning for God)
8.	*Ingluvies ventri* (gluttony)	*Abstinentia* (abstinence)
9.	*Acerbitas* (bitterness of heart)	*Vera largitas* (generosity)
10.	*Impietas* (wickedness, infamy)	*Pietas* (devotion)
11.	*Fallacitas* (lying)	*Veritas* (truth)
12.	*Contentio* (contention)	*Pax* (peace)
13.	*Infelicitas* (unhappiness)	*Beatitudo* (blessedness)
14.	*Immoderatio* (immoderation, anarchy)	*Discretio* (discretion, moderation)
15.	*Perditio animarum* (doom)	*Salvatio animarum* (salvation)
16.	*Superbia* (arrogance)	*Humilitas* (humility)
17.	*Invidia* (envy)	*Charitas* (charity)
18.	*Inanis gloria* (thirst for glory)	*Timor Domini* (reverence for God)
19.	*Inobedientia* (disobedience)	*Obedientia* (obedience)
20.	*Infidelitas* (lack of faith)	*Fides* (faith)
21.	*Desperatio* (despair)	*Spes* (hope)
22.	*Luxuria* (obscenity)	*Castitas* (chastity)
23.	*Injustitia* (injustice)	*Justitia* (justice)
24.	*Torpor* (lethargy)	*Fortitudo* (fortitude)
25.	*Oblivio* (oblivion)	*Sanctitas* (holiness)
26.	*Inconstantia* (instability)	*Constantia* (stability)
27.	*Cura terrenorum* (concern for worldly goods)	*Caeleste desiderium* (heavenly desire)
28.	*Obstinatio* (obstinacy)	*Compunctio cordis* (remorse, compunction)
29.	*Cupiditas* (craving)	*Contemptus mundi* (letting go)
30.	*Discordia* (discord)	*Concordia* (concord)
31.	*Scurrilitas* (scurrility)	*Reverentia* (reverence)
32.	*Vagatio* (vagabondage)	*Stabilitas* (stability)
33.	*Maleficium* (occultism)	*Cultus Dei* (dedication to God)
34.	*Avaritia* (avarice)	*Sufficientia* (satisfaction)
35.	*Tristitia saeculi* (melancholy)	*Caeleste gaudium* (heavenly joy)

SPIRITUALITY FROM DOWN UNDER

The soul affects the entire body with the power of the virtues or the weakness of the vices. Not even one biochemical reaction takes place in the body without the influence of the soul. Hildegard writes: "The soul rejoices in good, just as the body is delighted by delicious food. But when a person does something evil, this is as bitter to the soul as poison is to the body. The soul passes through the body just as sap passes through a tree. The tree is green through the sap, produces flowers, and brings fruits. But the fruits come to maturity only by the mercy of the grace of God that makes a person bright as the sun."

Overwhelming facts from modern medicine confirm Hildegard's impressive view of the body-soul relationship. A virtue such as love, compassion, trust, or hope positively affects wound healing, lowers blood pressure by decreasing the adrenaline blood level, calms the heart rate, and decreases life-threatening abnormalities such as poor digestion and migraine. The Christian virtues are the greatest healing powers when negative forces—depression, madness, anxiety, fear, rage, bitterness, arrogance, desperation, for example—are blocking the healing energy. Negative thoughts, emotions, and feelings are absolutely health destroying.

Hildegard's pattern of thirty-five virtues and vices can be used as a practical guide for meditation, fasting, and prayer.

For the first time in history the virtues and vices according to Hildegard's visions have been illustrated, by the painter Hans Meyers, professor of fine arts at the University of Frankfurt, Germany. Hildegard not only put the virtues and vices on stage and dramatized a dialogue, but also presented their typical thought patterns. The vices speak realistically and even fit very well in the modern world, while the virtues present their answers with heartfelt arguments.

Why are so many illnesses incurable today? Conventional medicine treats disease mainly on the organic level, neglecting to look at the psychosomatic causes. Diseases are a malfunction of the body and neither drugs, nor surgery, nor radiation can restore the body's deficiencies. It is impossible to solve an emotional problem with concrete remedies. Not even cancer can escape the problems of a disturbed soul. Cancer will keep returning until the negative psychic factors that caused the illness in the beginning are eliminated. It is extremely important to know that each problem is looking for a solution. Behind every negative force stands a positive spiritual healing force, and each weakness can be balanced by a spiritual strength.

As seen by Hildegard, the cosmic man and his thirty-five virtues or positive energies operate in harmony with the human soul, and the soul is permanently connected with the human body by way of the central nervous system. The skull and vertebrae hold the nervous system together and provide the location for nerve outlets. The spinal nerves follow the body segments to activate and stimulate the entire body and all its organs. Organs then send their life signals, via the nerves, back to the central nervous system.

According to anatomy, the vertebral cord has thirty-four vertebrae:

- seven cervical vertebrae
- twelve thoracic vertebrae
- five lumbar vertebrae
- five interconnected vertebrae comprise the sacrum
- five vertebrae comprise the coccyx

Altogether the thirty-four vertebrae plus the skull make thirty-five. These vertebrae, with their thirty-five spinal nerves, communicate with the thirty-five virtues and vices in our soul.

The discovery of this soul–nerve interplay in Hildegard's psychotherapy is one of the most important findings in the field, and enables us to detect the underlying risk factors for the soul-causing sicknesses. All we have to do is to examine the body, detect the organ defect via the *dermatomes* (head's zones), and bring the situation to the attention of the patient. Never label a patient by his vices or weaknesses: "You have colitis because you suffer from gluttony, bitterness, wickedness, lying, contention, unhappiness, immoderation, or depravity, and so on." Let the patient find out for himself: "Look in this region of the table of virtues and vices and ask, Is there anything of importance for me?"

It is sometimes more important to ask the patient about the condition of the mother's pregnancy when he was a baby in the womb. Was the mother under intense pressure from something or even contemplating abortion? The new baby feels everything, including love and rejection. The biography of a newborn human being is extremely dependent on the circumstances of pregnancy.

The next step could be a conversation with the parents to clarify the situation. Crying is helpful, as is any open-hearted word or gesture of forgiveness. As soon as the problem is understood and forgiven, the colitis can heal forever.

Our Social Relationship

The quality of our lives depends on our relationship with other people, with nature, and with God. We all search for good friendships, wish to enjoy a harmonious family, and yearn for the holy worship of the divine. A missing good relationship during our childhood can cause psychic deficiencies later in life. One third of the population in the Western world suffers from the inability to love. This disorder in daily life is characterized by a chaotic lifestyle, with cocky and egoistic behavior. These people cannot show compassion and can act only impatiently or angrily, and often lack a relationship with God.

Self-analysis

It is also possible to evaluate the psychosomatic risk factors by going through the table of vices and asking yourself: Am I a case of material love, petulancy, hard-heartedness, resignation, rage, and so forth? Do I need more love, discipline, modesty, compassion, trust in God, or patience? There is no human being without a need—that's what makes us human. Be pleased if you find your own imperfection, because there is a strong power behind every weakness. Become conscious of your problems. Practice fasting or meditate on positive virtues by repeating the mandalic words of the virtue until it goes into your heart, and you will be free of your addiction.

For twenty-eight vices, fasting can help you move in the direction of your virtue and enable you to make good decisions. The other seven imperfections or vices—love of the world, unhappiness, immoderation, lost soul, arrogance, inconstancy, and melancholy—can be changed only through spiritual prayer or meditation (for arrogance, sometimes you must go to a retreat alone).

Fasting is a universal source of life energy. Hildegard is actually saying that with the thirty-five virtues, the power of the universe is interwoven with us and everyone can receive an unlimited supply of the cosmic energy.

Rediscovery of Hildegard's Psychotherapy

Eight hundred years after Hildegard, Carl Gustav Jung, the great Swiss psychotherapist and a colleague of Sigmund Freud until their break, rediscovered—without knowing Hildegard's work—the virtues as images of the human soul, which he called *archetypes*. According to Jung, the archetypes are implanted in each human soul as in a storehouse of information.

Every psychic force has an opposing value: good and evil, love and hate, hope and desperation. Evil has the duty to show good; sickness leads to health; and an enemy becomes a friend. The goal in life is to bring both forces into balance. Don't kill the monster; he is extremely helpful in the journey to health and happiness.

Healing Is a Multidimensional Process

We must learn to enjoy the fact that we are multidimensional by nature. We must use the power of cosmic energy and of natural life energy in creation to heal and prevent diseases naturally. The spiritual nature of humans and their bioenergetic relationship to the universe is a mystery to today's medical profession, but is a key principle for healing in Hildegard's medicine. According to Hildegard, healing is a multidimensional process and occurs on four levels simultaneously:

- healing the physical body with natural remedies
- healing the soul with thirty-five positive spiritual forces
- cosmic healing with the energy of the four elements of the universe
- spiritual healing with the energy of the divine

HEALING WITH THE POWER OF THE DIVINE

"Therefore," writes Hildegard, "reflect upon your sickness, contemplate, and look for a physician before you die. He will give you a bitter remedy to heal you after he has diagnosed your disease. He will explore whether your intention to return and change your lifestyle is real or is labile and unstable like a breath of wind. After the investigation he will give you the wine of repentance and contrition to wash off the odor of your wounds. Then you will receive the oil of compassion to heal and regenerate.

"He will admonish you to take care of your health: 'Be careful and persistent in your repentance, because your wounds are serious.' Many people resist taking responsibility for their own mistakes. Some resist with great effort. But I stretch out my hands and turn their bitterness into sweetness. In this way they can experience repentance and live their lives to a good end in peace.

"Those ones who don't seek a physician and do not discipline their life do not ask for healing. They cover the smell of decay and erase the facts about their death, which they do not respect. They have no urge for healing and they despise the balm of compassion and the comforting words of salvation. They rush into death, because they do not look for the kingdom of God."

SPIRITUALITY FROM ABOVE, OR HEALING WITH ANGELIC POWERS

What shall we do? We can look for friendship with angels! Angels are friends and helpers of human beings in all their affairs. Our lives occur under the protection of the angels. Hildegard calls the protection forces *Militia Dei,* God's own military, which help us in moments of danger and also help us make the right decisions as we communicate with the outside world.

ILLUMINATION OF THE ANGELIC WHEEL

The angelic forces are essential for our fragile lives, which are protected from an immense, powerful security belt just as the cell nucleus, with the genetic code, is protected by the cellular membrane. The angelic protective force exists since the first day of creation because no life would exist without these powers. Hildegard makes the invisible innermost secret of life visible

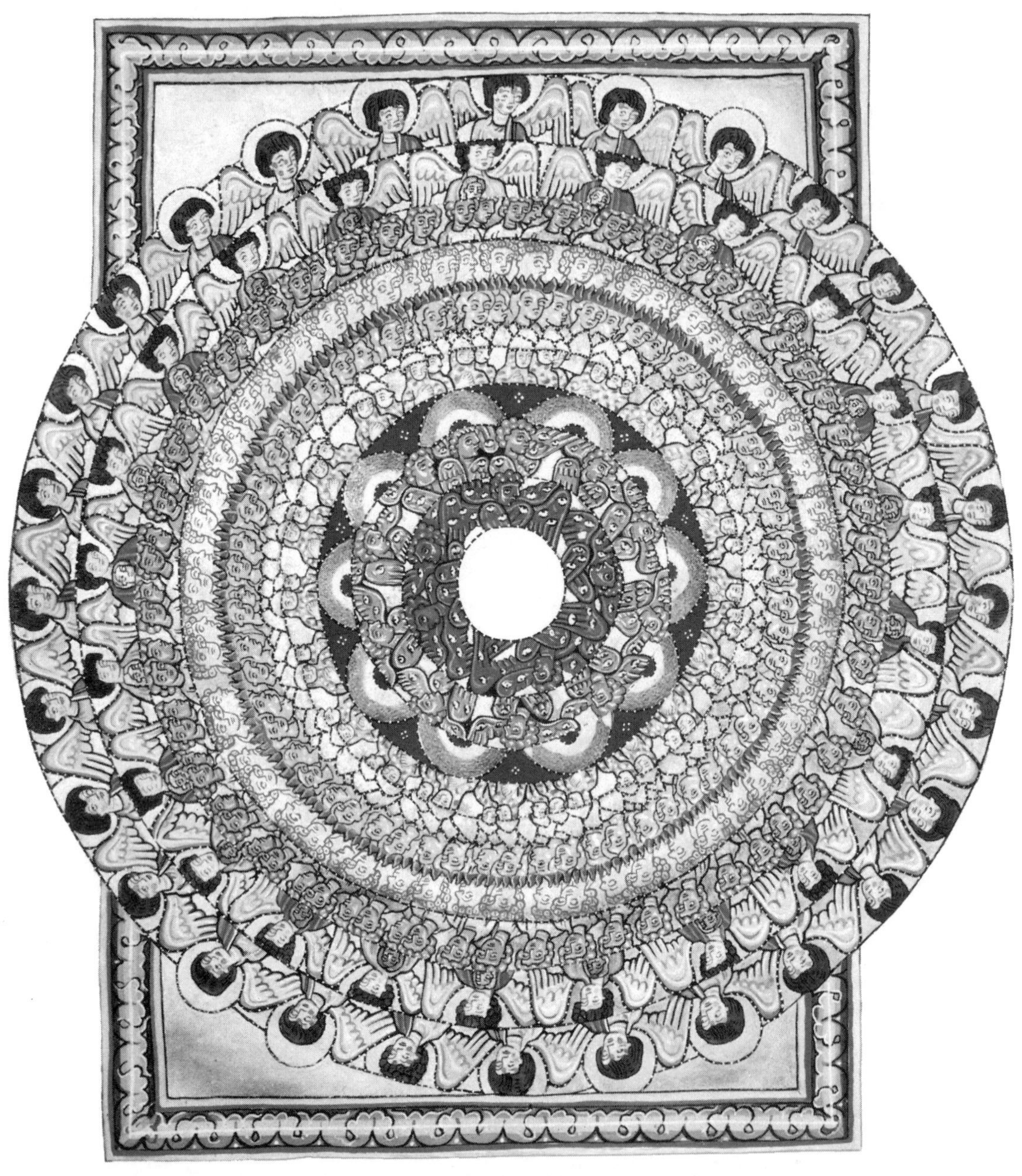

The Angelic Wheel. The nine concentric rings of angelic healing and protective forces maintain life on earth and in all creation. (*Scivias I,* Vision 6)

with the help of her microscopic vision, which shows nine concentric rings of angels protecting the white center of life.

Far from conventional belief, angels do not have wings and fly around like spiritual cosmic bats. They are strong spiritual healing forces who protect us from disease and provide us with spiritual values like the thirty-five virtues, which help us to make decisions. They represent moral standards to help us find our way and free us from the manipulation of other than God's will.

The angelic power field looks like the vibration of an electromagnetic field, which can intercommunicate between the micro- and the macrocosmos.

As we know, the universe is filled with vital bioenergetic fields, radiation, photons, and light, a complex network of cosmic energy to maintain life on earth and in all of creation. Day and night we are always connected with the higher-frequency energy system that empowers creation. No life exists without the energy of the sun and its radiation.

The American biochemist Melvin Calvin received the Nobel Prize for his discovery of the biosynthesis that Hildegard describes in her visionary words: "In the early morning during sunrise, the green of the earth and in the plants is the most powerful . . . during this time the plants inhale very much green just like lambs drink much milk."

Millions of green leaves absorb carbon dioxide from the air. Then, with the help of the sun's energy and chlorophyll, they produce carbon and oxygen to synthesize an abundance of plant protein, carbohydrates, vitamins, fat, drugs, aromatic fragrances, and plant colors like alkaloids and bioflavonoids, to name a few. This process is the basic principle for all nutrition on earth—without which life would be impossible.

ANGELS: GUARDIANS OF LIFE AND DEATH

The nine angelic rings encircle a white center into which we are invited to take our place because we are mirrors of God, his most beloved partners on earth.

Surrounding us on the outside ring are angels, representing the visible body. Underneath, in the second ring, are archangels: These symbolize the soul. The angels have faces like people and wings to expand their profound desire for the goodness of God. Their wings are not like those of a bird, but rather are wings to do the will of God quickly. They fly faster than the speed of light, just as do the thoughts of people, and represent the beauty of God's wisdom. Angels transfer the will of God to people and influence their actions.

ARCHANGELS: GUARDIANS OF WISDOM

Archangels are like an image of God's word shining in a mirror. They treasure the word of God most purely and know the deepest secrets of life. Their wings signify the intellectual power that is transmitted from God to humans.

The two rings of angels and archangels circle five other rings of angels arranged as if they were a crown. They signify the five senses. Body and soul are unified by the power of their strength.

VIRTUES: GUARDIANS OF THIRTY-FIVE HEALING POWERS

The first of the five senses represents the world of the eyes, the clear outlook to see heaven and earth simultaneously. Hildegard calls these forces virtues, "which ascend in the hearts of people" and move their feelings. The virtues continuously help people cast aside all the uselessness surrounding them so they can change the sorrow and stress of the world into joy and recognize the highs in the lows of daily life. Here the question rises: Is there a God? There is always hope as long as the question is asked and the answer is yes. When the question is no longer asked, then the answer, God's gift of repentance, falls by the wayside and the person "is cast down into death." We are invited to be awake and to see not only the visible world with our physical eyes but also the invisible world with the third eye.

POWERS: GUARDIANS OF ENERGY AND SALVATION

The next ring represents the powers that give strength to a person. It is interrelated with the world of the ears, the capability to integrate into the cosmic order through listening. "These forces reflect the beauty of the power of God. No weakness, nor death nor sin, can apprehend the serenity and beauty of the power of God, because the power of God is unfailing," writes Hildegard. Not only the outer ears hear, but also the inner ear listens to the soft voice whispering from the quiet, innermost parts of the soul.

PRINCIPALITIES: GUARDIANS OF SOCIAL JUSTICE ON EARTH

The principalities watch over those who exist as leaders and rule by the gift of God. These leaders are responsible to God and Christ and should always strive for the best interests of their people.

The third ring of principalities symbolizes the world of smell and fragrance, reminding us to have the right instinct in doing the right things at the right time.

DOMINIONS: GUARDIANS OF RATIONALITY AND COMMON UNDERSTANDING

The dominions help us to imitate the one who is the head and origin of all. Hildegard's important word *rationalitas* means the burning desire for reason and knowledge that leads to wisdom. This power is represented by our capacity to speak and influence others through the word. It also relates to our sense of taste and to the virtue of compassion. Hildegard calls compassion—the compassionate word—a *quasi medicina,* often much more effective than pills or any other medicine. And it "tastes" good!

THRONES: GUARDIANS OVER THE HEAVENLY SECRETS

The thrones of God glow in the dawn of the new day and are imbued with the mysteries of heavenly secrets that human weakness is not able to comprehend. Therefore, divinity itself bent down to humanity, touched it, and entered the body to show its one-ness with us. This is the fifth sense of moving and touching, because God's Son was touchable and lived visible among the people. The skin sense includes massage, sauna, baths, oil rubbings, hugging, and kissing.

CHERUBIM: GUARDIANS OF THE KNOWLEDGE OF GOD

The cherubim are covered with eyes that day and night look full of awe at God. Eyes always signify the knowledge of God, or *Scientia Dei,* as Hildegard calls it. In each eye is a mirror that reflects God's wisdom toward us so we can participate in God's creative knowledge. This knowledge includes that of healing and of prophecy as well as the charisma of the seven gifts of the Holy Spirit. The knowledge of God is revealed during meditation, which is practiced with the power of patience. The Latin word *patientia* is the virtue you learn when you exercise forbearance. Patience is a precondition for health and healing. Impatience makes us sick and angry and results in too much stress.

SERAPHIM: GUARDIANS OF THE LOVE OF GOD

The seraphim are burning as if they are fire. Hildegard writes that our sins burn in the fire of the seraphim. *Seraph* comes from the Hebrew language and means "burning, glowing," being close to God; indeed they circle in proximity to the innermost tenth place. The center is empty—it is the place for God but, miracle of miracles, it is also the place for you and me, because we are a wondrous miracle of God.

Friendship with the Angels

All the angels have wonderful voices and are accompanied by every type of music in order to glorify God. Everyone who sings and dances takes part in the joy and happiness of the angels, who are full of praise and harmony. Therefore, look for friendship with the angels and sing and dance to the symphony of the universe. Angels are our best helpers and guardians, not to be glorified like God, but to help us on our journey through life.

In Revelation 22:8–9, we find: "I, John, am he who heard and saw these things. And when I heard and saw them, I fell down to worship at the feet of the angel who showed them to me, but he said to me, 'You must not do that! I am a fellow servant with you and your brethren, the prophets, and with those who keep the words of this book. Worship God.'"

How do we become friends with the angels? A friend, a medical doctor in France, Jean-Marie Paffenhoff, heals his patients by calling the angels by name. In his book *Les Anges de votre vie* (not available in English) he recommends a very practical way to communicate with your angel: Call him by name. Angels can help only when you allow them to do so. The names of the angels are secretly hidden in the book of Exodus 14:19–21.

We journey through life in the shadow of a daily routine, traveling with a suitcase full of problems and conflicts in a spiritual flatland. When we begin to realize we are able to communicate with the angels, we discover our spiritual dimension.

The Cosmic Christ and the Power of Love

According to Hildegard, everyone has unlimited access to the positive virtues she sees centralized in a beautiful man, the cosmic Christ. He stands in the universe, his head in the highest summit of heaven, his feet down on the earth.

"I saw a man of such a height," she writes, "that he reached from the very top of heaven's clouds all the way down to the deepest depths. He stood there in this way: From his shoulders on he loomed beyond the clouds into the radiant ether. From his shoulders down to his hips another dazzling white cloud hovered around him, underneath the cloud layer mentioned before. From his hips to his knees an earthly atmosphere played around him. From his knees to his calves he was located in the region of the earth. His feet, finally, were submerged in the waters of the depths—however, in such a way that he still stood above the chasm" (LVM).

Man is a spiritual warrior and the virtues are his weapons. He is escorted by thirty-five beautiful women representing thirty-five virtues. Hildegard calls them *Militia Dei,* God's army, or protective forces. We can ask these forces to help us strengthen our immune system in our own daily fights against viruses and bacteria. Because we live in forgetfulness on earth, far from holiness, we have to remember that we are part of the cosmic Christ. We can remember through the help of spiritual means like prayer, meditation, and fasting. But we have to be active and apply the virtues in our daily life—there is no good unless we do that. Our active life of helping others should be combined with the inner work of prayer, contemplation, and meditation to create a greater world beyond the material world.

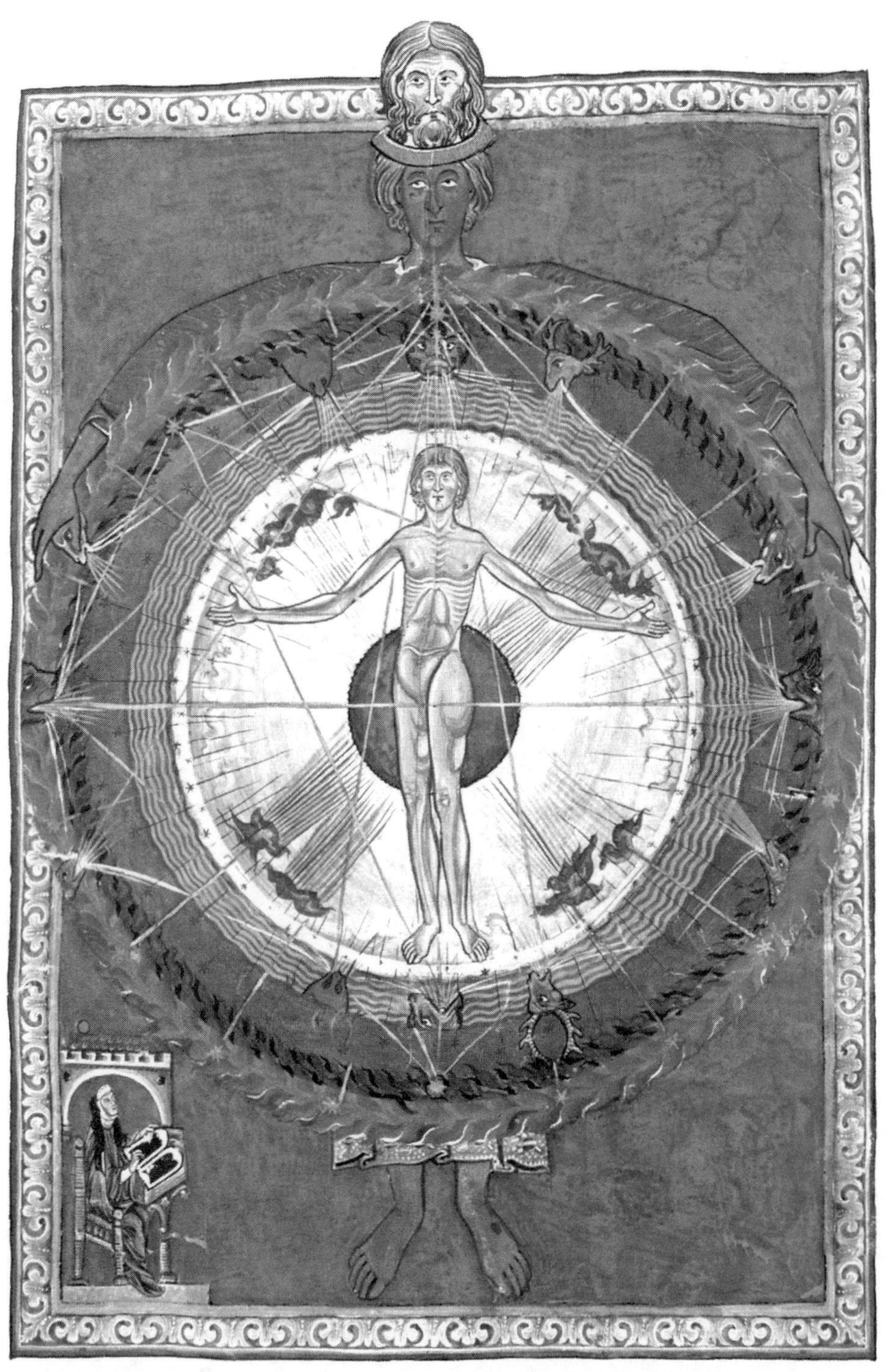

The Cosmic Christ and the Power of Love. God holds the entire universe in his hands.
(LDO, Vision 1)

THE COSMIC NATURE OF OUR SOUL

The body-soul psychotherapy of Hildegard is radically different from all other psychotherapeutic approaches, as it emphasizes the fact that the human soul not only is localized within human beings but is also interconnected with the entire universe. Our soul is free of time and space—eternal, infinite, all-powerful, and divine by nature. Healing is a process that can even go beyond personal healing, by healing others and healing our relationship with nature. No matter how sick and injured our bodies are, our souls are always whole, holy, beautiful, young, and healthy.

Anatomy of the Human Body and Soul

The image of the cosmic Christ is a magnificent metaphor for the human anatomy, where the visible body is the house for the invisible soul. The human soul operates with the help of divine energy, which is at the same time the building and defense force or the universe. *Humanity* and *cosmos* are two expressions from the same architecture.

The twin concept of the human soul and the universe hit Hildegard like a thunderbolt. When she turned fifty years old, she moved out of the Benedictine convent of the Disibodenberg, even against the will of her abbess Kuno, in order to build her own cloister up north on the Rhine River in Bingen. With the money of her family, she hired two hundred Cistercian monks, who were at that time the professional craftsmen for church and cloister constructions. Some of their buildings have survived and are still in use, such as the cathedral at Cluny and Maulbronn in Baden Württemberg, Germany. Hildegard took the blueprint of her cloister straight out of the Bible from Saint John's vision of the city of Jerusalem in Revelations 21:2.

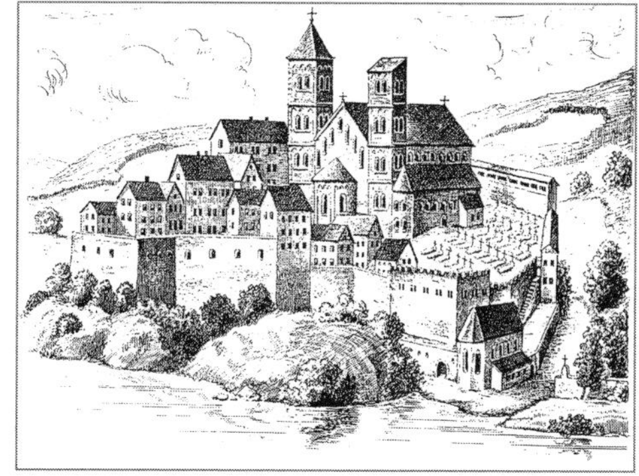

Illustration of Hildegard's cloister on the Saint Rupert mountain in Bingen

"I saw the Holy City, the New Jerusalem, coming down out of heaven from God, prepared as a bride beautifully dressed for her husband. . . . And he carried me away in the Spirit to a mountain great and high, and showed me the Holy City, Jerusalem, coming down out of heaven from God. The angels who talked with me had a measuring rod of gold to measure the city, its gates, and its walls. The city was laid out like a square, as long as it was wide . . ."

Hildegard's contemporaries were amazed; they had never seen anything like this. A woman built a cloister all on her own, without support from the church or the state. The beautiful cloister was erected on the mountain Saint Rupert, a saint for the pure and the sick. The area still has powerful vortex energy. The cloister was destroyed during the Thirty Years War, but the imposing church stood there in ruins until it was dynamited from the city of Bingen and removed to make place for the railroad.

Hildegard applied the blueprint of the city of Jerusalem in order to describe the performance of the human soul and body. The building blocks, towers, walls, columns, houses, and temples are comparable to different parts of our body, the home of our soul.

- The head is the center for the first seven virtues, which represent the seven senses.
- The body from shoulder to hips contains virtues 8–15, responsible for the digestive tract and its organs.
- From hip to knee is the center for forces 16–22. These regulate sexual energy.
- The region between knee and foot is the center for forces 23–30, which regulate the muscles of the hip and thigh.
- The foot and its five toes together make up the five virtues from 31–35, which are also responsible for all other powers: 31 for the seven powers of the first group (seven scurrilities); 32 for the eight powers of the second group (eight vagabonds); 33 for the seven powers of the third group (seven magic forces); 34 for the eight powers of the fourth group (eight avarices); and 35, a guiding force for all other forces.

The Language of the Soul

The soul speaks to the body via the neurons of the autonomic nervous system in order to exchange information and keep the body healthy and alive. Neurons communicate with each other through electrochemical energy and special chemicals called neurotransmitters. Information travels very quickly within different types of nerve cells, some at a speed of 120 meters per second—equivalent to 268 miles per hour!

The cranial nerves bring information from the sense organs to the brain; others control muscles, glands, and internal organs and functions such as the heart, lungs, digestion, and sexuality. The optic nerve, for example, controls vision; the olfactory, smell; the facial, taste; the vagus nerve, sensory perception and motion as well as autonomic function of digestion and heart rate.

The spinal cord is the main pathway for information connecting the brain with the body. The spinal cord is protected by the spinal column, which is made up of bones called vertebrae. Most vertebrae are flexible; however, some in the lower part are fused, containing thirty-five segments: seven cervical, twelve thoracic, five lumbar, five sacral, five coccygeal, along with one—the cranium, which surrounds the brain.

The first cervical vertebra holding the skull is called the atlas. Atlas is one of the Titans from Greek mythology. He was turned into a stone after a fight with Perseus and had to carry the sky on his shoulders for eternity. In the same way, the atlas vertebra must carry the weight of the entire head.

The thirty-five vertebrae correspond to the thirty-five forces called the thirty-five virtues and vices of the human soul. The soul controls the function of the body via the autonomic nerve system by sending out information to the spinal cord through the spinal nerves. The nerve fibers enter the spinal cord left and right through a dorsal horn that looks a bit like the wings of a butterfly.

The Autonomic Nervous System: Bridge between Body and Soul

The autonomic nervous system within the vertebrae communicates with the body by sending out impulses to the heart and to the glands. It also controls the functioning of the circulatory, respiratory, digestive, and urogenital systems.

It controls blood pressure, blood circulation, heartbeat, body temperature, and the gastrointestinal system, especially the functioning of intestinal microflora; the acid, enzyme, and mucus secretion of the digestive organs; and the hormone supply. Also under its control is the immune system, a complex army of organs, cells, and molecules that can activate more than 100 million immune cells in order to fight against bacteria, viruses, and other enemies of our environment. Health and disease are heavily dependent on the proper functioning of this system.

The autonomic nervous system operates with two hands that have opposite effects. The sympathetic nervous system stimulates the heart, dilates the bronchi, contracts the arteries, and inhibits digestion during action in a fight-or-flight situation. The parasympathetic nervous system does the opposite during rest and sleep.

In the past we thought the autonomic nervous system operated by itself like an automaton, or robot, without regard to our will. Today we know through countless studies what Hildegard revealed eight hundred years ago: that lifestyle affects the so-called autonomic nervous system. Negative feelings such as hate, anger, and fear as well as positive emotions like love, compassion, hope, and joy exert a strong influence on the autonomic nervous system, causing either health or disease.

Dr. Larry Dossey's book *Healing Words* and Dr. Herbert Benson's *Timeless Healing* outline the clinical research that demonstrates what Hildegard already knew—that prayer, contemplation, and meditation positively affect healing. Consider these examples:

- a wound that heals naturally over time
- blood pressure that goes down
- the LDL (harmful) cholesterol level that goes down; the HDL (good) cholesterol count that goes up
- the heartbeat that normalizes
- the immune system that rallies to keep out infections and to destroy any germs that get in, including cancerous cells

We know from Hildegard that our soul consists of thirty-five positive healing virtues that stay in balance with thirty-five negative risk factors, the so-called

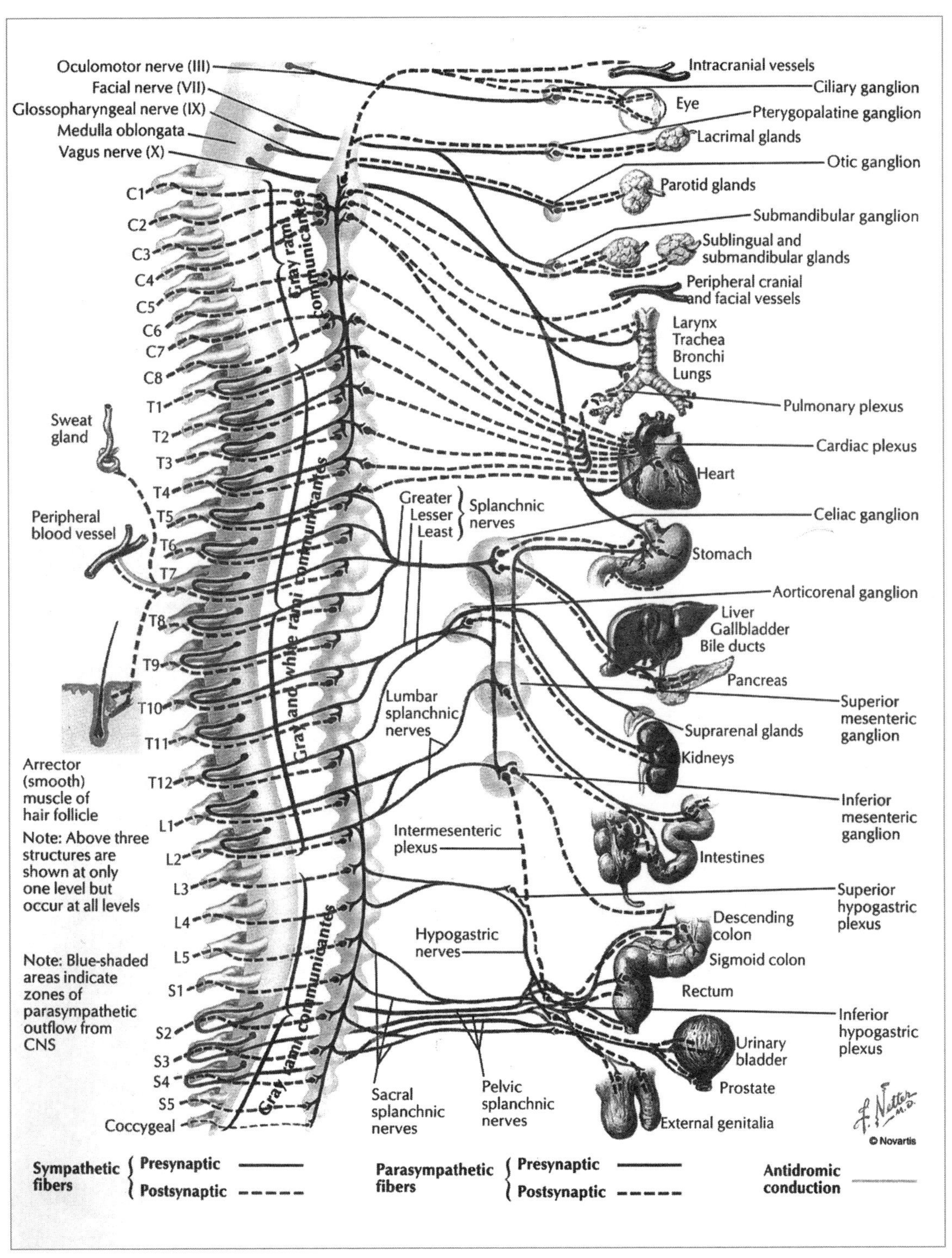

"Autonomic Nervous System," Microsoft @ Encarta @ Online Encyclopedia 2000.
Illustration of the Autonomic Nervous System (*Atlas of Human Anatomy*, Frank H. Netter).
This source has been used for every organ relationship in the text.

vices, which are detrimental to our health. Life is a process of constant learning to balance body and soul and keep them in a working relationship. Hildegard's healing art supports us in our efforts.

Ordo Virtutum: The Dance of Life with Virtues and Vices

Healing requires holistic understanding and knowledge of how the soul operates. Hildegard gained this knowledge through her visions, which are more than human intelligence or experience with the five senses—they are the voice of divine wisdom. She describes the forces of our divine souls, along with the positive behavior that increases energy and the negative influences that weaken it.

The health and well-being of our bodies depend entirely on the energy status of our souls. In order to heal the body, we must always consider the performance of body and soul. Every dysfunction of the body requires healing of the soul, and healing of the soul requires activating the power of the divine energy represented by the thirty-five virtues, or healing forces.

Hildegard dramatized the interplay of body and soul in a musical dance performance called "Ordo Virtutum." The human soul journeys through life and collects her experiences in the school of Earth. The master of hell drags the human soul through thirty-five life-destroying learning experiences leading to spiritual blackout and weakness. Sooner or later this results in life crises—which are absolutely necessary to awaken the divine power of the soul. This awakening requires learning from the depths: through sickness, the death of a loved one, the collapse of a business, perhaps.

On the other side, according to the law of attraction, we can also learn from the thirty-five positive healing forces. Love attracts love, discipline attracts a healing energy, and hope creates peace of mind. It depends on our decision: Do we choose the way of the visible or of the invisible world? The ultimate question is: Which road do we take—the path of hate or the path of love? Both ways can lead to the health of our souls. The negative way is more painful, dangerous, and full of poison. Only strong personalities can survive, but they may be covered with scars even as they achieve the blessings.

In order to study the relationship of body to soul, we can experience the energy that flows from the thirty-five positive forces such as love, peace, hope, and joy or the energy loss that results from the thirty-five vices such as greed, anger, brutality, and depression. All the virtues are uplifting and energizing and lead us into an atmosphere of relaxation, peace, and healing. The corresponding vices are life-destroying, bringing low energy, fatigue, and a loss of immune strength.

The play of the thirty-five virtues and vices has three acts. First we get involved with the arguments of two opposing powers, such as love of the visible material world against heavenly love of the inner invisible world of the divine. Every word is potent and powerful in our brains, which are very sensitive. A word can kill or heal; it can be a poison or a remedy. The virtues use healing words. These words are a wake-up call to the soul to activate spiritual healing energy. Sometimes they speak in affirmations, as in exalted prayer to create superior healing power. Positive thoughts deactivate negative energy and activate the healing power of our souls. This healing power is at the core of our well-being. Anima, the soul, is torn between the virtues and vices; she loses her white robe and moves into the darkness.

In the second act of the spiritual play we see the physical dysfunction that results from the negative influence of the vices. Negative emotions such as anger and hate, despair and greed have low energy and cause blackouts and organic damage to the body. In her vision Hildegard sees symbols of physical dysfunction such as fire for inflammation, bugs and worms for infection, and ditches with gas and sulfur for indigestion and damage to the intestinal flora. Anima, the lost soul, moves farther and farther from the virtues and deeper into the darkness.

The final act recommends spiritual means to heal the soul and liberate it from negative behavior or addiction. Fasting is the universal remedy for twenty-eight spiritual problems; the other seven require spiritual healing exercises such as prayer, living in isolation, and physical training.

The purpose of Hildegard's spiritual psychotherapy is to achieve personal well-being and the healing of body and soul, which requires knowledge of the thirty-five virtues and the thirty-five vices and the healing power of the divine soul. Anima, the soul, remembers her original home and returns, receives her white robe once again, and is reunited with the virtues in salvation.

Chapter 3

The Eastman

The man turns around in the universe and looks east toward the rising sun. Here, in the east of the universe, we see seven strong, divine building forces emerging with the sunrise. The first is heavenly love; she is the energy that brings the entire universe into being and keeps it alive. The second force is discipline. The Greek word for *discipline* means "cosmos," and the order of the cosmos keeps the universe together. The third power is respect, admiration, and friendship—understanding that the entire universe is a living organism working harmoniously. Compassion is the fourth foundation of the universe, the power that creates mutual love and understanding. The divine victory, number five, is the power on which the universe is built with confidence and trust in God.

The arrangement of the universe needs two more forces, patience and at-one-ment, for its proper function. Patience brings peace of mind and serenity; at-one-ment acknowledges that the universe operates through the power of God.

THE FIRST SEVEN POWERS AND THE SEVEN SENSES

Our lives before life comes from the love of *Amor caritatis*. The moment of conception is the beginning of our biography and responsible for the health of our nervous system and the harmonious performance of our seven senses. Optimistic, healthy children are born when conception occurs in perfect and mutual love. *Amor caritatis* is the orgasmic power of love transmitted in the moment of conception with a combination of perfect humors and hormones.

Amor caritatis is the Latin expression for erotic love and mutual appreciation transmitted from man to woman in the moment of orgasm. When *amor* and *caritas* combine, they draw on universal and earth forces to create a new prenatal energy within the embryo. This prenatal energy strengthens our ability to attract the spiritual forces from the universe to sustain our health and well-being. Under these conditions, the energy of love and dignity during embryogenesis creates healthy children with a disposition to love, discipline, modesty, compassion, trust, patience, and worship of God. The first seven virtues of our lives are counterbalanced by the seven negative vices, which regulate the functioning of the seven senses.

1. *Amor saeculi* (material love)	*Amor caelestis* (heavenly love)
2. *Petulantia* (petulance)	*Disciplina* (discipline)
3. *Joculatrix* (love of entertainment)	*Verecundia* (decency, tact)
4. *Obduratio* (hard-heartedness)	*Misericordia* (mercy, charity)
5. *Ignavia* (cowardice, resignation)	*Divina victoria* (God's victory)
6. *Ira* (anger, criminality)	*Patientia* (patience)
7. *Inepta laetitia* (inappropiate mirth)	*Gemitus ad Deum* (sighing to God)

The first seven virtues inhabit a tower of the city of Jerusalem with two parts: one with five arches for the first five values (1–5) and one with two arches for the next two forces, 6 and 7.

The seven virtues are all beautifully dressed women representing the feminine or spiritual part of humanity. The vices are mostly men with animal bodies, symbols for the masculine or earthy part of our souls.

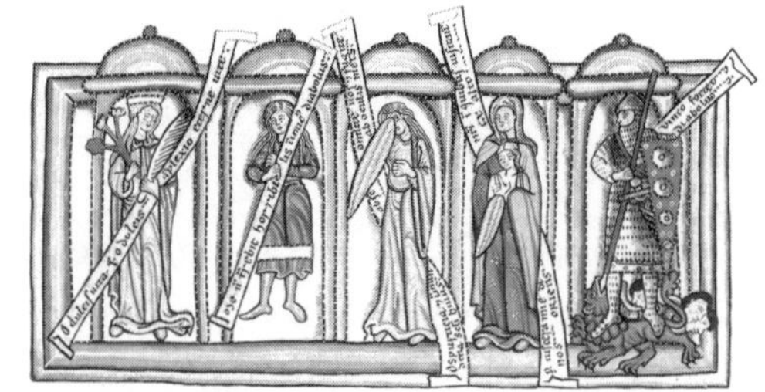
Illumination: The Tower of Jerusalem

The tower represents the region of our souls with the seven senses. The senses are the gateways that communicate between our inner world and the outside, macrocosmic world. Whatever happens in the organism has a cosmic influence and what occurs in the cosmos affects the organism.

The seven forces are responsible for the health and the harmonious interplay of all seven senses, which are in communication with the autonomic nervous system and the first seven cervical vertebrae.

1. *Amor saeculi* **Material love**	*Amor caelestis* **Heavenly love**
Love of the visible world	Love of the invisible world
Love of material values	Love of spiritual values
Love of the ego	Love of your real personality
Love of your outside image	Love of your divine soul
Spiritual blackout	Spiritual power

Crystal Therapy

Gold topaz wine is the appropriate therapy.

Place a gold topaz in a shot glass full of wine for 3 days. Moisten the eyelids once or twice a day for 5 days with the wet gold topaz. Continue with the same procedure, using new wine, as often as necessary, but for at least 3 months. This helps cataracts, glaucoma, and poor vision.

THE EYES ARE WINDOWS OF THE SOUL

Have you ever seen a soul? Hildegard writes: "The eyes are the windows to the soul." All you have to do is look into the eye of a friend and watch the miracle of the eye, how it reflects the power of the soul. The eye reflects the universe: the black pupil the moon, the iris the radiant sun, and the sclera the firmament. The eye reveals love, anger, anxiety, health, sickness. The eye sees the visible world; and the inner eye sees the invisible world.

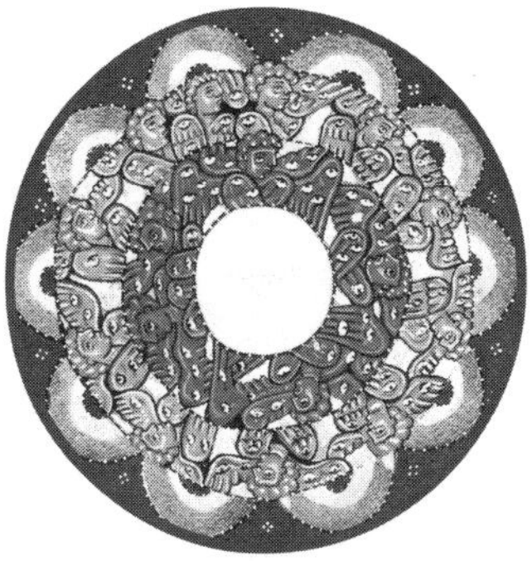

All of us can meditate until we see with the inner eye, a beautiful opportunity for the soul. The golden square of our souls, or divine eye, is packed with many eyes to see the world's inner reality. The virtue Fear of God wears a dress covered with eyes to see the wonder of God and the miracle of creation day and night. These eyes know the glory of God and heavenly love. The red circles of seraphim and cherubim have eyes on their wings. They reflect the burning fire of love, they know about God, and their red color shows divine love infusing humanity. The purpose of our seeing is to make the invisible world visible.

SEEING WITH THE INNER EYES, HEARING WITH THE INNER EARS

Hildegard was a master of audio-vision and made the invisible world visible in her illuminations. Throughout her life she acquired knowledge and wisdom through vision and intuition, which is knowledge beyond the knowledge we gain through experience with our five senses. It is the knowledge that inspires every artist, such as Bach and Mozart in music and Michelangelo and Picasso in art, as well as Shakespeare and Twain in literature.

Hildegard has only one source, the divine wisdom and guidance through God, which she reveals in her books. She opens her inner eyes and ears and speaks:

"I saw a very great light from which a heavenly voice spoke and said to me: 'Speak and write those things not according to yourself or to another person, but according to the will of the One who knows everything, who sees everything, and who arranges everything in the secret depths of the divine.'

"In the year 1141, when I was forty-two years and seven months old, a burning light coming from heaven poured into my mind. Like a flame that does not burn but rather warms, it inflamed my heart and my body, just as the sun warms us with its rays. Suddenly I was able to understand books, the Psalms, the Gospels, and the Old and New Testaments. . . . I received the vision not in dreams, asleep, or mentally disturbed, neither with my own eyes and ears, nor in faraway places. I received my visions awake, alert with a clear mind, with inner eyes and ears of my spirit according to the will of God" (SC, foreword).

In similar words Hildegard explains her audio-vision in *Book of the Divine Works:*

> It was in the year 1163 of the incarnation of our Lord, during the schism from Rome under the emperor Frederick I, the red beard, when a voice came from heaven, speaking to me:
>
> "Transmit what you see with the inner eyes and ears of your spirit for the benefit of humanity. . . . Write this down, not according to your heart, but rather according to my will. . . . This vision is not your invention and not conceived by another person, but rather I have all of it planned from the beginning of the world."
>
> Everything I had ever written in my earlier visions and learned later on I recognized was under the influence of heavenly mysteries. My body was fully awake and I was in my right mind. I saw it with the inner eyes and heard with the inner ears of my spirit. I experienced my vision never asleep nor in ecstasy. I received my vision rather from celestial secrets without any human influence. (*Book of Divine Works,* foreword)

THE IMAGE OF MATERIAL LOVE

Love of the world is represented by a naked man grabbing for the blossoms of an apple tree. When he grabs the blossoms, the tree collapses and so does the man.

Harmful Words of Material Love

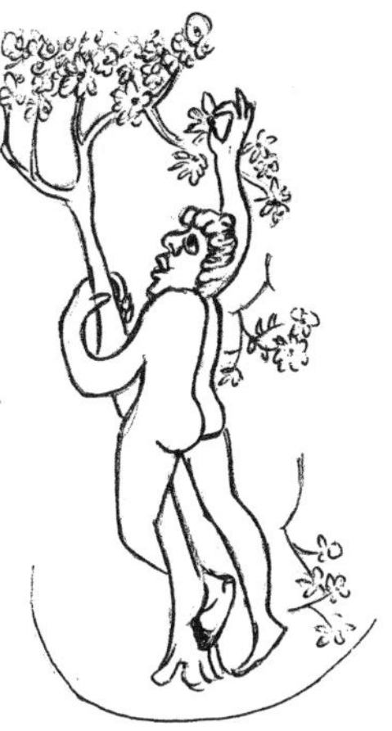

Love of the Material World speaks these words:

"I possess all the resources of this world. Why should I fade as long as I am fit and beautiful? Should I run around like an old buffoon while I'm flowering at the peak of my youth? Should I close my eyes to the fascination of the world? As long as I can, I will enjoy the beauty of this world and will grasp it with delight. I know only the world around me and no other life" (LVM).

Hildegard's vision of the naked man and the falling tree reminds us of the contemporary global player of our times and his insatiable greed. Money buys everything and anything—sex, power, science. The lover of money and possessions becomes addicted to the material world. His hunger for more, greater, bigger can never be satisfied. One wish stimulates another. With both hands he grabs with lust for the many fruits of the world and destroys them in the moment of fulfillment. Both he and the fruit tree break down and collapse in the darkness. The downfall of the lover of materialism goes along with ruin, destruction, energy loss, weakness, and finally sickness and death.

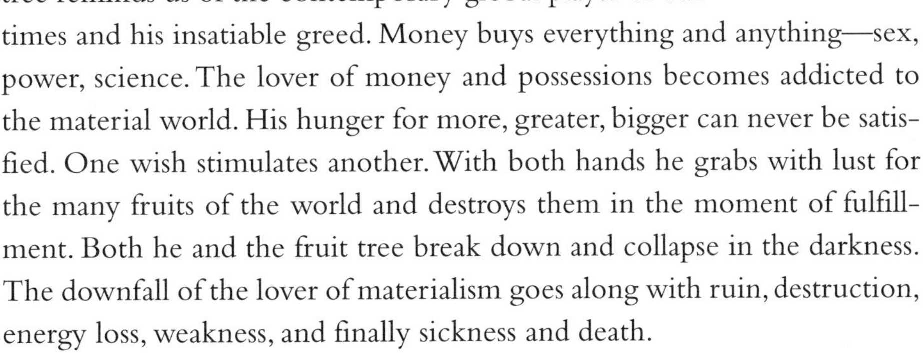

It is a proof for the justice of the universe that wealthy people in the Western world have to spend all their money to treat the so-called incurable illnesses caused by an excessive lifestyle and an overabundance of food. Eighty percent of those sicknesses could be prevented if only we changed to a reasonable lifestyle and a proper diet! On the other hand, the same incurable illnesses are absent from the poor people in the Third World. Clothing and money as well as incurable sicknesses were absolutely unknown to the Aborigines before the white man discovered Australia.

Sooner or later the accumulation of material wealth leads to personal or social crises such as autoaggression, suicide, and sexual or emotional violence. Not until the love of material things breaks down either through sickness or the loss of his possessions will he wake up. Many people choose to learn through pain and breakdown instead of wisdom and spiritual enlightenment through heavenly love. But no matter what we choose—the spirituality from down under, learning through crisis, or learning from wisdom—there are golden healing words that transform love of the material into heavenly prosperity.

Healing Words of Heavenly Love

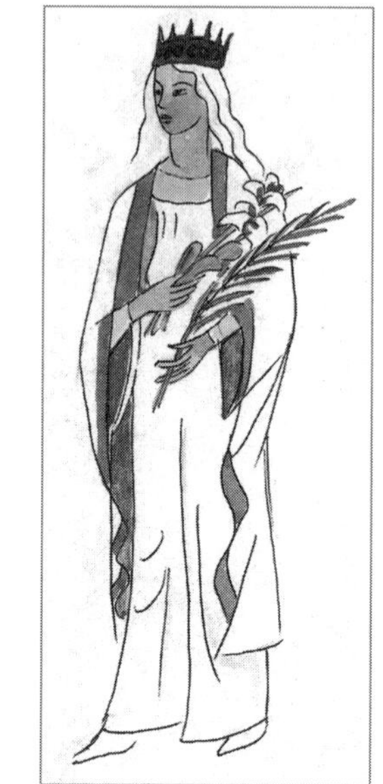

Heavenly Love speaks:

"You are insane if you search for life in a little bit of ashes. Real life is young and beautiful, and never ages. Why are you not searching for the real life, which never fades from the beauty of the young or even disappears in the most meaningful and wonderful time of growing older? You need clarity and light! Once your vision is clear, you will notice how your life is being spent shoveling in the dark like a worm underground. Life is short from one end to the other, and eventually you decay like hay. You will disappear into the depths with all your questionable property.

"I am filled with heavenly harmony and love the real life. I attack people who destroy it. I reflect all virtues, so that the faithful awaken and become visible. You follow a dark track and the work of your hands goes to hell" (LVM).

The world offers us only temporary wealth; God gives eternal treasure. The greatest present of the invisible God is his Son, the visible image of the invisible God. Heavenly love begins when you see this image in yourself and in your neighbor.

> O sweet life and sweet embrace of eternal life and blessed happiness in which there are eternal rewards. You are so delightful that I am always satisfied with the inner joy that is in my God. (SC III, vision 3:1)

We all live from the life power of God, which is eternal, endless, omnipotent, and empowering. He loves you and me as a lover does his beloved.

He endows us with wisdom to receive the gift of understanding and awareness and the power of positive thinking. Positive attracts positive; love attracts love! God is our partner, and when we wish for good, we receive it. When we wish for evil, the devil brings ruin and destruction according to the cosmic law of attraction. Writes Hildegard, "Whatever we do good or bad comes back to us good or bad."

Organ Relationship

Material love and spiritual blackout are related to the pathology of the nervous system in the region of the cervical vertebrae, especially the atlas (C1). The atlas controls the nervous system of the five senses, the facial muscles, and the blood circulation of the heart and arms. (See Frank H. Netter, *Atlas of Human Anatomy*, plate 153, page 45.)

In Hildegard's vision, Material Love causes sicknesses such as arthritis, rheumatic fever, myalgia, and neuritis.

> I saw two fires burning, one with cold blue and another with ruby red flames squirming with many worms. Some were biting others with sharp, knifelike teeth. Many people who idolized the material world were burning in both flames, although most were in the ruby red flames of infection, due to their heavy involvement with financial and material wealth during their lifetime. (LVM)

"Others with a lesser interest in the business world suffered only trouble and pain. The hypocrites, who openly condemned what they did in secret, had immense pain from the bites and from the fire. Others who had slightly damaged the world were stung from the bugs only until they learned their lesson."

Meditation on Heavenly Love

Love is the top priority of our generation. Each of us strives for love but still suffers from its lack. The reason for this paradox is a misunderstanding of the basic nature of love: The more we demand, the less we get. Love disappears when we take it by force.

None of us has the power to make someone else love us.
But we all have the power to give away love.
—RABBI HAROLD KUSHNER

The more we give, the more we receive. Heavenly love is the result of a harmonious relationship among my neighbor, my God, and myself. Love of the world, on the other hand, grabs for material wealth. This world collapses in the moment of usurpation. Hildegard illustrates this by a muscular man pulling down apples out of a tree. Man and tree are engulfed in misery, because the fruits are being taken by force.

Love of the world blocks the way to the invisible world, the realm of the spiritual world. "I tell you my secret," says the fox to the little prince. Only the heart can see good; the essential is invisible for the eye!"
—ANTOINE DE SAINT-EXUPÉRY

Spiritual Healing

A sickness can be therapeutic when we read and understand the message of its symptoms. Patients having trouble with their eyesight or suffering from rheumatic arthritis can look for the psychic background of these diseases, especially during fasting. Cultivate love of the invisible world through simple fasting with fennel tea and bread. Wear clothing made from coarse material that scratches and follow the guidance of a friend with whom you can talk about the love of God. Physical activities such as walking and taking a sauna are also helpful.

Read, pray, and meditate on Psalms 119:18, 121;
I Corinthians 2:9–10; and II Corinthians 4:16–18.

2.	*Petulantia*	*Disciplina*
	Petulance	**Discipline**
	Disorder, chaos	Order, cosmos
	Out of control	Under control
	Out of bounds	In regulation
	Malevolence	Kindness, tolerance
	Stressful lifestyle	Harmonious lifestyle

Crystal Therapy

Jasper is the appropriate therapy.

Cut jasper to an olive-shaped piece that will fit in the ear canal. Attach it to a silver chain for removal. Lick the jasper and put it into the ear for 15 minutes once or twice a day. This helps in cases of deafness caused by ear infection or catarrh.

The Greek word for *discipline* translates to "order of the cosmos." Chaos is the opposite, and that is exactly what petulance is all about: confusion and disorder through extravagance, diversions, clamor, and hullabaloo. Nature works with everlasting rule: "Everything created by God is connected with one another."

The Ear: Health Center of the Body

Everything that enters the ear has a healing or sickening effect on the body. Our brains and especially the autonomic nerve center, which regulates the housekeeping of our body, are very sensitive to sound, words, music, and noise. The ear is a gateway between the world around us and the inner world.

Sound energy travels through the air and enters the ear. The eardrum (tympanic membrane) receives the sound waves and transports the signals via the hearing bones into the labyrinth of the inner ear to the cochlea, the real hearing center. The sound waves are changed here into electromagnetic frequencies that stimulate the brain. The brain waves cause either relaxation or excitement and can be traced visibly by an EEG.

These brain waves are divided into four different rhythms: beta, alpha, theta, and delta. Beta waves are associated with normal waking consciousness; alpha and theta are increasingly relaxed states; and delta waves indicate deep sleep. These brain waves influence every cell in our bodies and thus can heal or damage the physical body. Relaxation waves lower blood pressure, slow down the heartbeat, release stress from the immune system, and prepare to fight viral and bacterial infection and kill cancer cells.

The gastrointestinal system is especially sensitive to good music. Baroque music is often played during dinner to create a pleasant atmosphere.

Sound works not only on the body but also, even more powerfully, on the soul, where it can activate its divine energy. Spiritually, sound transports the voice of God to the inner voice of the soul by the power of the Trinity. God the Creator creates with his word. The creative power of the word travels physically via sound waves to the ear through the power of the physical God, Jesus Christ. The power of God's spirit moves into the brain and causes a reaction, a mood change, an awakening, a call that can instantaneously change our lives and heal. This is the reason that words can heal or regulate body functions. Everybody who prays or heals with words of love or compassion takes part in this divine creative process.

Hildegard explains that especially the liver and body metabolism are influenced by what we hear. The noise level is sometimes so unbearable that the inner ear shuts down in order to restore and regenerate. Many people experience this at loud concerts or during stressful periods as a hearing insult that can cause deafness or chronic tinnitus. It is possible to therapeutically heal the liver by listening to good music.

Words have the power either to heal or to kill. The diagnosis "You have cancer; you are a hopeless case and there is nothing that can help you" is like murder. The interferon level of the immune system can plunge to zero, causing the cancer to accelerate. This is poison to the body and causes depression and cynicism. Petulance is pictured as a stray dog.

Harmful Words of Petulance

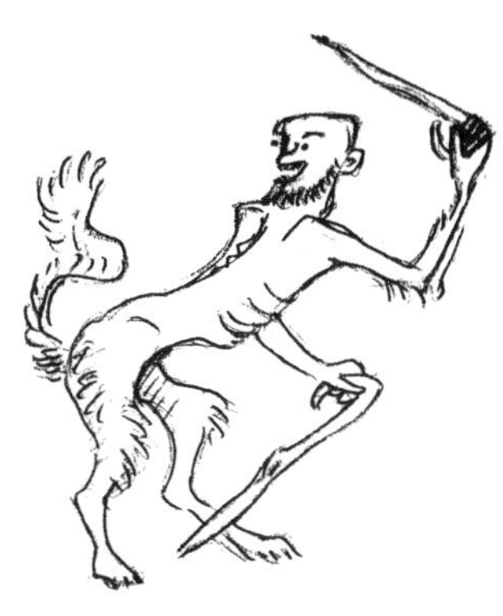

Petulance speaks:

"Hello, fans, let's enjoy ourselves as long as we're alive. Why not be riotous and enjoy entertainment as long as we have something to laugh about? The human soul likes a blast if you bring it into vibration with the right harmonies. I don't want to live like a bum and walk around like death. Let's be merry as long we have something to laugh about" (LVM).

Rock, pop, and techno prove that music can be a drug that hypnotizes people. The fact that music can make us aggressive and pull out of the brain the last molecule of adrenaline has had terrible consequences for both society and the younger generation. I have treated several young people with hearing trauma after a techno night. It is no wonder that the number of deaf and neurotic people is rising.

Healing Words of Discipline

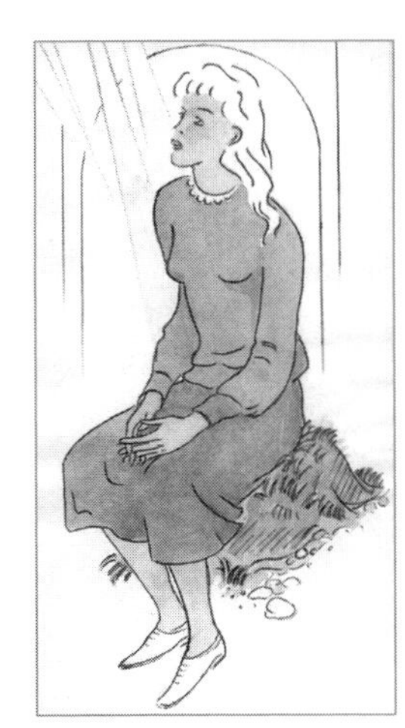

Out of the chaos comes the yearning for a new life full of stillness and joy. Only harmony and discipline create an atmosphere of peace of mind. Discipline speaks:

"You're a silly clown. You act like a tornado with your filthy manners. You jump on people like a dog and make them stupid and foolish. You offer them what they desire. You hurt people's hearts with your dirty jokes. You are the trickster who pretends to live in accordance with the rules. You lead people by the nose and change them into morons.

"I carry the golden belt of wholeness and I inspire dignity, excellence, and honesty. I am invited to the wedding celebration of my king and appear with great joy. I hurry to the wedding celebration beautifully clothed in justice" (LVM).

All amusement is fleeting and its end is followed by the blues. What counts is the stability of Discipline:

> Neither the horrible enemy Satan, nor a hostile person, nor this era will scare me away from the teachings of God, in whose vision I stand all the time. (SC III, vision III, 3:2)

Organ Relationship

Petulance is related to the pathology of the nervous system in the region of the cervical vertebrae, especially C2, which controls the sense of hearing. The nerves here are also responsible for the facial muscles and the blood circulation of the head and arms. (See Frank H. Netter, *Atlas of Human Anatomy,* plate 153, page 45.)

Hildegard sees in her vision of petulance and chaos symbols like fire and worms causing inflammation and pain. These are probably sicknesses related to rheumatic fever, muscle pain, and neuritis, as in the rheumatic pain of the muscles and nerves of the back and feet or attacks of the sciatic nerve. "I saw a gigantic fire and a dark cloud that made the fire almost invisible," Hildegard writes. "In the fire many worms squirmed with wild alarm and noise. People living in stress and chaos felt as if they were suffering in the burning fire. They could barely breathe anymore because of the sticky air. They were burning on their feet and all over the body due to their chaotic and extravagant lives."

Meditation on Music

There is no doubt that music has healing power that affects the human soul, working on the physical body in order to release stress, regulating the breath and heart rhythm, and energizing the immune system. We can use music to change mood, increase creativity, and open a window to the harmony in the universe. The entire universe is related to music and sound. That's why Hildegard calls her musical visionary work *Symphony of the Harmony of Celestial Revelation.*

For Hildegard, music is much more than we understand today; music is the most perfect symmetry and balance of the macro- and microcosmos, heaven and earth, God and humanity. Music is the way we can immediately and powerfully change the way we feel and think by bringing into alignment the inner and the outer world. The human soul itself is "symphonically tuned."

What is it that makes Hildegard's music so extraordinary? Hildegard removes the barrier of the previous Gregorian norms and brings us into the realm of the cosmic symphony—her music reveals the resonance of the celestial order.

Music for her is closely related to the science of mathematics. The Boston mathematician Dr. Pozzi Escot shows by computer analysis the hidden geometrical structure in Hildegard's music and the relationship between the architecture of the Gothic cathedrals and her chants (*Sonus: A Journal of the Investigations into Global Musical Possibilities,* vol. 5, no. 1, p. 14).

Hildegard's music is perfectly composed in accordance with the ratio of the Golden Mean—that is, a musical expression of audiovisual harmony. If we sing Hildegard's antiphons, we participate in the geometry that links heaven and earth. The visible expression of her songs reveals, for example, an architectural facade of the cathedral at Chartres.

Music can be quite therapeutic. Hildegard explains that music changes the nature of body and soul so powerfully that healing energy flows in every cell of our bodies. Music can also in a few seconds release rage and pain or increase energy by recuperating body and soul *(omnia recuperant).* Music can open our senses and thinking, cleansing everything *(omnia purificant).* Music creates a oneness in the inner and outer world and makes everything holy, whole, and healthy *(omnia sanctificat).*

In summary, music regenerates, purifies, sanctifies, and harmonizes everything instantaneously, both body and soul *(omnia continent).* Music sings heavenly and earthly songs simultaneously, bringing together God and humanity in harmony.

Spiritual Healing

Petulance can be transformed into a disciplined life by fasting in moderation, eating simple foods, and drinking beverages without alcohol. It is also helpful to speak with a friend about discipline and to practice the six golden rules of Hildegard.

1. Your food will be your remedy.

2. Your remedies should be natural, not chemical or genetically manipulated drugs.
3. *Ora et labora:* You should meditate and rest as much as you work.
4. Keep exercise and rest in good balance.
5. Purge your blood and humors with bloodletting, cupping, and intestinal cleansing.
6. Purify your soul with Hildegard's psychotherapy and fasting.

Read, pray, and meditate on Psalm 34, with its emphasis on ears and hearing; John 5:24–30; Romans 10:14–18; and the following verses about discipline: Proverbs 1:7, 10:17, 12:1, and 15:32, and Hebrews 12:5–11.

3. ***Joculatrix*** **Love of Entertainment**	***Verecundia*** **Love of Simplicity**
Joker	The respectful person
Carelessness, recklessness	Care, discernment
Impoliteness	Politeness
Tactlessness	Tact
Immodesty	Modesty, discretion
Rudeness	Courtesy
Disregard, dishonor	Cherishing, esteem, honor
Derision, condescension	Intuition, perception

Crystal Therapy

Jasper helps hay fever and sinusitis.

Cut a jasper into an olive-shaped stone to fit in the nose and attach a silver chain for easy removal. Lick the jasper, then place it in each nostril for 15 minutes.

THE POWER OF SMELL

"Whoever gets really angry should take roses (*Rosa damascena* oil) and less sage (*Salvia officinalis* oil) and smell this in the moment of anger. Sage comforts and roses bring joy and happiness."

Rose-Sage Oil

This perfume is Hildegard's most powerful fragrance against the destructive mood of anger.

Mix 5 ml (1 teaspoon) of almond or olive oil, 4 drops of rose oil, and 2 drops of sage oil and store in a dark bottle. Use it as a perfume, body oil, or simply sniff it.

The smell of a lily *(Lilium candidum)* is also very powerful, as the scent "gladdens the human heart and raises the spirit to create right thoughts." Hildegard praises lily oil for its effectiveness in supporting intelligence, thus leading to concentration and wisdom.

Lily Oil

It's simple to make your own lily oil.

Take a large Madonna lily and cut it into pieces. Place them in a clear glass bottle filled with 100 ml of olive or almond oil. Cover the bottle and let stand for ten days on a sunny window sill. Remove the plant material and decant the oil into a dark bottle.

Just as lilies clear the spirit, the smell of lavender *(Lavandula angustifolia, L. officinalis)* clears the eyes and is a potent antiseptic. Lavender can prevent viral infections and even strengthen the body during precancer and cancer. Because lavender is one of the less toxic oils, we can massage the whole body in times of serious illness. But care must still be taken by people who are allergic. They should first apply 1 drop to the body, rub it in, and wait five minutes. Don't use lavender if you notice a red spot. We can make our own lavender oil using the procedure for Lily Oil, above.

Fennel *(Foeniculum vulgare)* is 100 percent good for our health and mood. As a carminative, it helps our digestion by creating good humors and blood. Gas and putrescent smells are naturally eliminated, thus producing a pleasant body odor and sweet breath. One liter of fennel tea daily is better than any chemical deodorant against body odor during stress and bad digestion.

Hildegard praises the herb for its ability to combat depression and suggests using fennel oil as a natural tranquilizer and tonic for muscular energy, especially after sports and convalescence from a severe illness: "People who suffer from melancholy, take fennel oil and apply on temples, nape of the neck, breast, and the entire body, especially rubbing the area around the stomach and solar plexus—the depression will disappear." There is a great feeling of harmony, peace, and freedom after the fennel massage.

Fennel Tea

This tea makes a powerful deodorant.

Boil 3 tablespoons of fennel seeds in 1 liter of water for 3 minutes. Strain and discard the seeds. Drink a cup of the tea several times a day.

Fennel Eye Remedy

Fennel also makes a marvelous remedy for eye inflammation, such as conjunctivitis.

Soak a handkerchief in 1 cup of fennel tea. Fold the cloth and use as a compress on the eyes several times a day. Symptoms will soon disappear.

These examples of aromatherapy show that essential oils and herb scents and fragrances are extremely helpful remedies and even strong mood changers. The effectiveness of odors is based on the spontaneous interplay of the nose with the brain. Odor molecules in minute quantities reach the sense of smell, which is located in the olfactory organ on each side of the nasal cavity, just below and between the eyes. The chemical odor produces in the receptors of this organ signals that are transmitted directly and immediately to the limbic system in the brain, which is the center of emotions, behavior, and memories.

The nature of the sense of smell allows it to identify good or even dangerously spoiled food, sharpen the appetite, and facilitate digestion. The male perspiration gland can secrete a smell (called androstenone), when the man sweats, that smells somewhat unpleasant but acts like an aphrodisiac stimulant for women. Oil of neroli creates an atmosphere of pleasure and even triggers sexual attraction. Other perfumes like fennel and lavender oil calm the nervous system in times of stress, anxiety, and even depression.

Perfumed oils of herbs and spices, scented barks, and resins have a long tradition in both medical and religious use. The Egyptian art of embalming used cloves, nutmeg, and cinnamon as natural preservatives for the human body and as companions for the journey to eternity. The scent of roses is a symbol of holiness and immortality. The sweet smell of roses comforted the women when they came into the tomb of the resurrected Jesus.

When the tomb of the evangelist Saint Mark was opened in the year 500, a cloud of rose scent wafted over the entire city of Alexandria. Today the remains of Saint Mark rest in a reliquary in the main church of Mary and Saint Mark in Germany on the island of Reichenau in Lake Constance. The church is directly across from my office and many sensitive people can feel very strong vortex energy coming from the church over the lake.

Chemical smells in strong concentration have quite a different effect: They can create an atmosphere of aversion and even stink like feces or the sex organs of a goat or of a musk ox. But the dilution of such odor in very low concentration causes just the opposite, an extremely pleasant smell that can stimulate sexual desire. Such fragrances are used today to attract the opposite sex and to encourage shoppers in a department store to spend their money with great pleasure. In this respect, smell can be an invitation to love and to be joyous or a trickster fooling and seducing us.

Petulance leads to the love of entertainment and pleasure. Love of Entertainment is a monster with a big nose like a clown's. The nose is like a hook or magnet leading people astray by attraction or enticement.

Harmful Words of Love of Entertainment

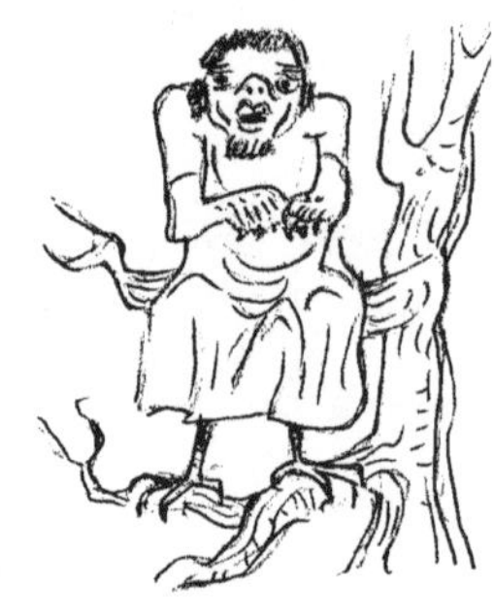

Love of Entertainment speaks:

"It's better to amuse myself than to suffer from melancholy! Games and diversions are not immoral! Heaven is ecstatic with every creature. Why shouldn't I have fun too? Nobody would love me if I ran around moping with the blues. I'm not stupid. I will dance and joke and make everybody happy. Did not God create the air and the beautiful scent of blossoms to attract woman and man?" (LVM).

Healing Words of Love of Simplicity

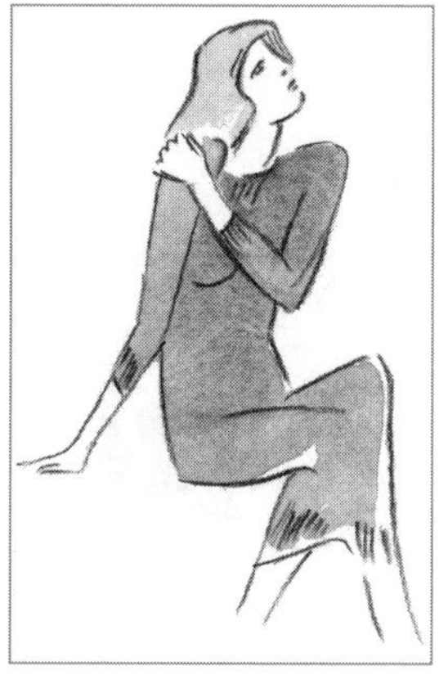

Love of Simplicity responds:

"You are a voluptuous celebrity, addicted to your own enjoyment. You are a man-made dead noise. You behave simultaneously like an animal and a man. You are more a dying than a living creature, as you are only looking for more attractions. You are vanity; the laughter of fools is vanity. Your work is only noise and smoke. You behave not like a human being but more like an animal, mostly like a rotten monster.

"I turn red with shame and look for protection under the wings of God's love. God leads me in the mysteries of his holy books. The divine influences my life. I look with pure, innocent eyes and understand God's will, that which you in your foolishness ignore" (LVM).

Television and other media make fools out of men and women. The show must go on. It is no joke! The joker, the entertainer, the showmen are the best paid people in our society. Teachers of wisdom are beggars. God's gift of wisdom is free. Even the emperor Augustus joked in the moment of dying: "Friends, applaud, the game is over!"

In almost modern words Love of Simplicity cries:

> O filth and morass of this age, hide yourself and flee from before my eyes,
> for my friend has been born of the pure Virgin Mary. (SC III, vision 3:3)

Organ Relationship

Love of entertainment and shamelessness, on the one hand, and love of simplicity, decency, tact, and modesty, on the other hand, are all related to the sense of smell. The nose can smell the atmosphere around us. It is very sensitive and perceptive about what is good for us and what stinks.

Love of entertainment is related to the pathology of the nervous system in the region of the cervical vertebrae, especially C3, which controls the sense of smell. The nerves here are connected to the trigeminal nerve, which is responsible for facial muscles. About 70 percent of all odors stimulate the trigeminal nerve receptor and cause side effects to the face, teeth, mouth, and scalp. (See Frank H. Netter, *Atlas of Human Anatomy,* plate 153, page 45.)

Spiritual Healing

The spiritual healing of love of entertainment occurs during fasting when we avoid luscious and rich food like fatty cheese, strong alcoholic drinks, animal meat, sausage, and eggs. The tactless joker can also be helped by contemplation and meditation.

The following Bible passages are particularly effective against shamelessness: Psalms 115:1–13 and 139, especially verse 6; Song of Songs 1:1–4; and Philippians 1:9–11.

4.	***Obduratio***	***Misericordia***
	Hard-heartedness	**Compassion**
	Lack of mercy	Goodness
	Indifference	Thoughtfulness
	Couldn't-care-less attitude	Goodwill
	Insensitivity	Sensitivity
	Rudeness	Kindness
	Heartlessness	Sympathy

Crystal Therapy

Diamond water is needed for crystal therapy. It prevents stroke and arteriosclerosis and is also helpful for regeneration after stroke.

Place a diamond (cut or raw) in a pitcher of water for 24 hours. Use at least 2 quarts of diamond water a day for everything you drink or cook.

Hard-heartedness is a leading cause of hardening of the arteries, stroke, and heart attack. The thick smoky form of Hard-heartedness has no limbs, only great black eyes and a sharp tongue. The image of God disappears in a human with no compassion.

Harmful Words of Hard-heartedness

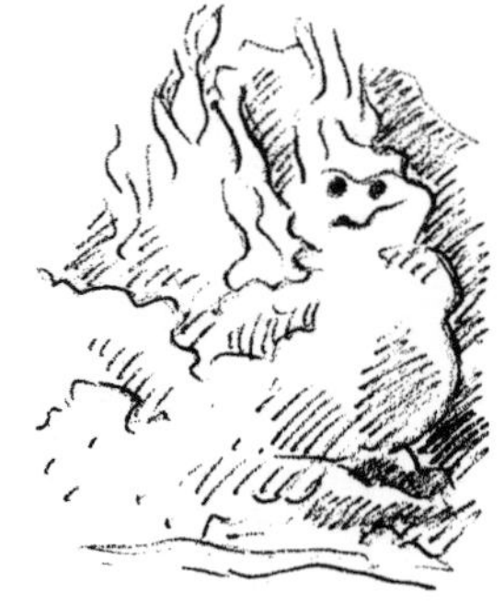

Hard-heartedness speaks:

"I did absolutely nothing; therefore, I'm not responsible. I couldn't care less. Why should I worry? Nobody looks after me—that's why I won't stand up for anybody anymore. God, who created everything, should care for his own creation. There is no advantage to me when I care for others. If I had compassion for all the trouble of the world, I would have no more time for myself. I know only myself, and everybody else should care only for himself" (LVM).

Healing Words of Compassion

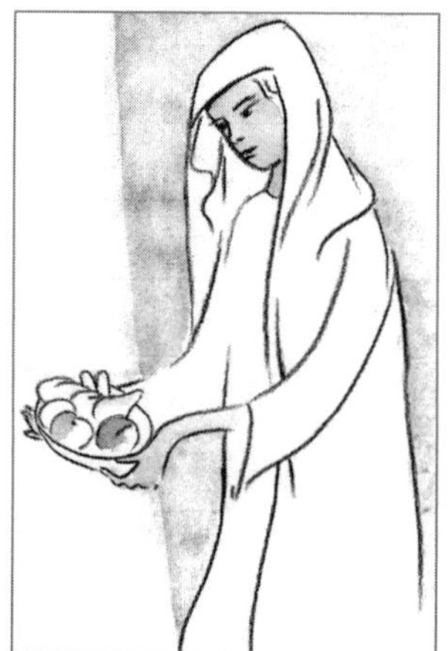

Compassion is a powerful force that can transform the hardest criminal. Mercy or compassion possesses healing energy—*quasi medicina*—just like a good remedy. Compassion speaks:

"Oh, stone, what do you say? The herbs and plants on earth flourish and exude their beautiful fragrance. One precious stone shines on the other. The whole creation yearns for love and affection. Creation serves humankind and gives its best for free, like a present. You are cruel and thoughtless, a dark smoke, bitter and toxic.

"But I am like dew, a strong life energy *[viriditas]* and a sweet remedy for everyone. My heart is full of love for everyone who needs my help. I have existed since the origin of life, when the great fiat—"let there be . . ." set creation into being. You were excluded already. My eyes always see whatever is necessary. I feel responsible and heal the sick, as I am a mild remedy. My compassion is sincere, whereas you are bitter smoke" (LVM).

Healing is a result of compassion. Performing "ear diagnosis," which means taking time to listen with the entirety of your heart, shows someone you care.

LEX DIVINA: THE LAW OF DIVINE COMPASSION

What shall we do? What is the purpose of life? Questions about a meaningful and happy life have always moved humanity. A lawyer stood up and asked Jesus, "Teacher, what shall I do to inherit eternal life?" And Jesus said to him, "What is written in the law?" And he answered, "You shall love the Lord your God with all your heart, with all your soul, with all your strength and with all your mind, and your neighbor as yourself." Do this and you will live.

The missionary physician Albert Schweitzer, who shared almost his entire life with the blacks in Africa, advised the same thing in his words to American medical students: "I don't know how your life will be, but I know that the only ones of you who will be happy are those who serve others."

The virtue Compassion also says:

> I always stretch out my hand to foreigners, to the needy, to the poor, to the weak, and to those who groan. (SC III, vision 3:4)

Practice Compassion

- "I was hungry and you gave me food!"—good, natural, organic food, not gourmet or genetically grown food.
- "I was thirsty and you gave me drink!"—natural beverages, not harmful soft drinks or "light" drinks.
- "I was a stranger and you sheltered me!"—in good natural houses of wood or stone, not of cement and poured concrete.
- "I was naked and you clothed me!"—with good natural cloth, not synthetics.
- "I was sick and you helped me!"—with natural remedies, not harmful chemicals.
- "I was in prison and you came to me!"—in the form of compassion to free me from my own prison of addiction, obsession, and bad habits.

The Seven Deeds of Compassion

To live in accordance with universal wisdom, the so-called seven laws of compassion *(Lex Divina),* means to be fully integrated and in harmony with yourself and with everyone else in a higher energy that sustains life as part of a divine plan.

The seven deeds of compassion provide us with basic spiritual guidelines for what it means to be human. If we respect these rules, we maintain excellent health, eat only healthy foods, drink good water, live in a natural environment, and open our eyes to the spiritual gifts we already have within us.

In denying these guidelines, our life simply will be attached to the material things of the outside world. But life teaches that not even all the money and possessions of the world can give us the inner joy that comes from inner gifts like real love, friendship, and a solid, loving family. We reach such spiritual richness by practicing and remembering the laws of compassion each and every day.

THE GUIDELINES

1. Eat natural food, in contrast to manipulated or genetically engineered food. If someone was hungry, would you feed him poison? When cows eat infected feed, they acquire mad cow disease. Do you like fast food, which causes food allergies, or hormone-doped meat that causes breast, colon, or prostate cancer? Do we have to produce genetically manipulated vegetables that disturb the intestinal flora and cause allergies?

Life is sustained with natural foods containing everything we need for our bodies. One of the oldest grains is spelt, which was a basic food in the Orient, Egypt, and all over Europe. Spelt has the oldest tradition in human nutrition and helps prevent or cure civilization diseases. If we eat the old, nonhybridized spelt, we have all the proteins, carbohydrates, fat, minerals and trace minerals, and vitamins for daily life. Due to its concentration of basic minerals, spelt neutralizes the acidity of black bile, which is responsible for the excess acidity that causes autoimmune sicknesses.

2. Drink fresh water instead of chemically enriched diet drinks. If somebody was thirsty, would you give him chemicals to drink, which harm his health? Phosphoric acid in light drinks leaches calcium from our bone material, making them brittle and prone to breakage; refined white sugar causes cavities and yeast infections. Children who consume a lot of sugar can become hyperactive and aggressive. Many drugs —antibiotics, cortisone, estrogens from birth-control pills and estrogens given during menopause, chemotherapy during cancer treatment, aspirin and other anti-inflammatory drugs—are recycled into our water supply. In addition to this, many agro-chemicals such as pesticides, insecticides, and herbicides pollute our drinking water and thus cause severe allergies and cancer. Drink only fresh springwater or water from natural sources.

Drinks for Compassion

- filtered water from the depths of a lake
- distilled water
- fresh-pressed juices from organically grown fruits
- herb tea from fennel, green tea, and rose hips
- spelt coffee
- spelt beer or natural barley beer
- wine with a few drops of water, or quenched wine (see page 241)

---

3. Wear natural clothes instead of synthetics or textiles with harmful chemicals. Our skin is influenced day and night by cosmic energy from the sun, moon, and stars. Life would be impossible without this energy. Traditional clothes like animal skin, leather, silk, and wool protect against heat and cold by being interconnected with the cosmos. Many native peoples believe the power of an animal—a bear or a buffalo, for example—transfers to those who wear it. Clothing represents, therefore, the second skin.

In addition to this tradition, various cultures used textiles whose origin is plants, like linen and hemp *(Cannabis sativa),* which are extremely healthful. Columbus could not have discovered America without hemp sails, which absorb almost 30 percent humidity. Cotton sails would tear immediately. The first jeans were made from hemp until the cotton industry invented the story about hemp being a psychotropic drug. Skillful textile makers go back to hemp because of its antiperspirant properties.

In contrast to this, chemical antiperspirants such as tributyltin (TBT) in sports jerseys are extremely poisonous, and cause burning of the skin and contact allergies. Other textile additives are azo dyes, which decay during sweating and become carcinogenic amino acids. Textiles from Third World countries contain agrochemicals like DDT and lindane as well as pentachlorphenols as preservatives. All these chemicals are very toxic and are implicated in allergies, cancer, and the weakening of the immune system. Use textiles from organically grown plants or animal skin without toxic additives.

4. Live in ecological houses instead of sick buildings. The Greek word for house is *oikos,* as in *ecology,* the art of living in a natural environment. Our skin is our biological house and it is connected to the cosmic environment.

Living in a concrete house full of toxic chemicals makes us chronically ill, the so-called sick-building syndrome. Patients are sick from the air they breathe, contaminated with hundreds of chemicals from paints, solvents, adhesives, and foam; industrial furniture and carpets smell like formaldehyde; internal and external electro-smog pollutes our brains. Sick-building syndrome is responsible for headache, sleeplessness, chronic fatigue, depression, loss of memory, and early nerve breakdown.

Many chemicals destroy the immune system, the result being auto-aggressive diseases. These diseases, which can destroy every organ and every cell in our bodies, include cancer, gastritis, colitis, hepatitis, pancreatitis, nephritis, neurodermitis, allergies, and asthma. Most people who suffer from these conditions are classified as neurotic and receive more toxic drugs.

Especially in danger are children in schools built under high-voltage wires. It is also dangerous for men and women to work in offices with air-conditioners—these recycle bacteria and viruses from other people.

Toxic Chemicals

The following chemicals cause skin allergies as well as liver, nerve, and kidney damage: asbestos; dioxin (TCCD); expodin-resin in glue, cement, and adhesives; formaldehyde in solvents; furanes from synthetics and adhesives; polychlorinated benzene (PCB) in foam and paint; trichlore ethane in cleaners; vinyl chlorides in floor covering; and xylole in solvents.

Those who feel sick should move into biologically sound houses built from natural materials like wood and clay and treated with natural paint and solvents. Avoid too many high-tech installations like microwaves and mobile phones with high frequencies that grill your brain. Install a night switch to regulate electricity for a better sleep.

---

5. Heal naturally without chemotherapy that uses poisonous drugs. According to a 1994 Toronto University report, modern medicinal drugs are among the leading causes of diseases and death. In addition, drugs destroy and pollute the environment. Heal in accordance with natural remedies in harmony with nature and human beings.

6. Live free and independent, not addicted. Western society today is hostage to its own habits and addictions. The hunger for more has no limits, nor has addiction—whether it be to food, alcohol, nicotine, coffee, money, work, sex, or entertainment. Desire triggers more desires, and will lead eventually to addiction and the inevitable path into prison. On top of this, we lose our free will and happiness. As soon as the kick is over, we look for more satisfaction.

Because we are born to be free and independent, we need a higher power to unlock our jails. Life starts when the old hang-ups die, when we let go of all possessions that kill life. Too many cars, clothes, bank accounts, and so on capture our life. The Aborigines had no clothes and no money; possessions were not important. Instead they liked to dance and sing, to tell stories and paint. Are we ready to open our prison and let go of our daily enjoyable poisons?

7. Bury the death disposition, obsessions, and addictions. All cadavers are toxic and must be buried so that new life can arise. Some tribes of New Guinea used to eat their own dead and developed *kuru,* a brain disease similar to mad cow disease, a terminal illness. When the Nobel Prize–winner Dr. Carolus Gadjusek discovered the pathogen similar to a prion, he recommended the tribes stop eating their dead and the kuru disappeared. New life starts when old life dies and the dead are buried. The original power of rebirth offers a new beginning. In the same way, we can use every sickness to point us anew toward salvation. Rebirthing poverty opens our eyes to wealth. Slavery turns into freedom. By flipping the coin called obsession we find discipline and self-control on the other side.

The seven deeds of compassion will guide the spiritual traveler through life. These deeds are easy to accomplish and can create prosperity in all areas of our society. Once we practice this art of living in our daily life, we learn to open our eyes to the true spiritual life. As soon as we let go of our compulsions and hang-ups and practice the seven laws of compassion, we become free and ready for real life. Liberation from our modern pseudolife is an essential condition for genuine life and pure happiness.

Organ Relationship

Hard-heartedness is related to the pathology of the nervous system in the region of the cervical vertebrae, especially C4, which controls the sense of taste and the tongue. (See Frank H. Netter, *Atlas of Human Anatomy,* plate 153, page 45.)

In her vision of hard-heartedness, Hildegard sees symbols of arteriosclerosis as fissures and cracks, as in vasculitis. We can even recognize clogging of the arteries with plaque and embolism.

> I saw a deep, dried-out fountain with boiling tar in the ground. A great cleft was visible and fiery smoke and glowing worms welled up from under the ground. Sharp, fiery knives were swinging in the wind down in the fountain. Those people who were hard-hearted during their lifetime had to sit at the bottom of the fountain. They were scared to burn in the fire. They suffocated from the fiery smoke, because they had separated themselves from God in their maliciousness. The worms attacked the people because of the pain they put on others. Fiery knives cut the people because of their lack of compassion. (LVM)

Meditation on Compassion

Compassion is therapeutic; Hildegard considers compassion a remedy. The celebrated Swiss physician called Paracelsus (Theophrastus Bombastus von Hohenheim) rationalizes: "The only reason for healing is compassion." Healing takes place when the right word is spoken at the right time. Such a word is in the liturgy for communion: "Lord, I am not worthy to have you come under my roof; but only say the word, and my servant [my soul] will be healed" (Matthew 8:8).

The spoken word, according to Hildegard, is a symbol of the presence of the divine in three qualities. The word is creative like the Creator; it is physically transmitted to the ear and is understandable like Jesus, who spoke to his people; and it causes a reaction in our spirits like the spirit of God, which fires and activates us. The power of a word is based on the language we speak—our mother tongue, from the Latin *lingua,* or "tongue."

During healing, we have to watch our tongues. There is a rule in medicine that if you don't have the diagnosis and you don't know a remedy, don't speak. A diagnosis—especially a wrong one—puts a curse on the patient and can harm and even kill. For example: "You have cancer. There is no a cure. You have to face the fact that, according to the statistics, you have only one year to live." This diagnosis would be a shock to anyone, and absolutely deadening. Such a shock causes the interferon level of the immune system to go down and the cancer then takes over. The diagnosis is like a voodoo ritual that brings about death. Words are powerful, and our brains are sensitive to words. The oldest church in Germany is the St. George Church, located on the island of Reichenau across from the Hildegard Guest House. In the altar room is the famous cowhide with this proverb: "No cowhide can hold the words that foolish women gossip all day long, Blah, blah, blah." Be careful with your words, for a word is like an arrow: Once you have fired it, you cannot take it back. Sometimes it is better to listen and to be quiet than to speak. Compassion helps love grow in the heart.

Spiritual Healing

Spiritual healing of hard-heartedness takes place during severe fasting with only soup, fennel tea, or hot water for at least a week and sauna therapy with brush massage according to the instructions of the fasting master.

For Bible passages exuding compassion, read, pray, and meditate on Nehemiah 9:5b–31 and Psalms 51, 103, 116, and 145.

5.	***Ignavia***	***Divina victoria***
	Cowardice	**God's victory**
	Resignation	Confidence
	Frustration	Trust in God
	Despair	Faith in God

Crystal Therapy

The amethyst is helpful for skin ailments such as warts, bruises, exotosis, old-age spots, and benign lumps in the breast.

Lick the amethyst and rub it in circles on the skin several times a day.

Cowardice tends to block healing energy and gives rise to chronic skin problems. In Hildegard's vision, most of the coward's body is boneless like that of a worm. The head has a rabbit ear, because desperation is a result of gossip and an evil tongue. Despair lives in a negative atmosphere of talking all day long about horrible events. The "Isn't it awful?" approach costs a lot of energy, destroys the immune system, and leads to an incurable state. The coward is the ultimate yes-man or yes-woman, like a boneless worm without any personal position or opinion, always afraid to hurt somebody. The coward is also the typical "poor me."

Harmful Words of Cowardice

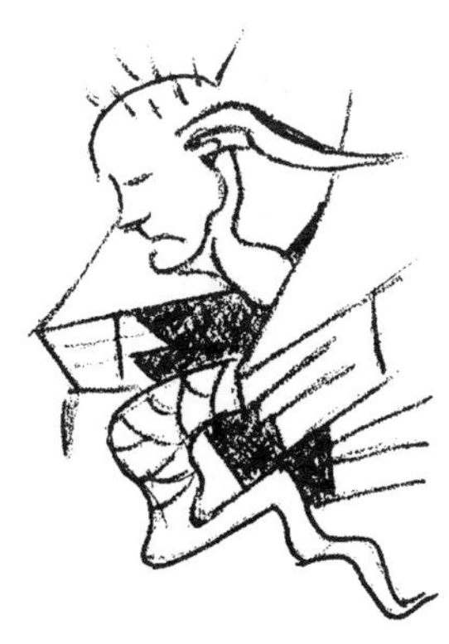

The Coward speaks:

"I don't want to hurt anybody, because I need help and consolation. I would lose all my friends and my existence if I were to get in trouble with them. I care only for the rich and for people in power, not for the poor and the saints, who are of no advantage to me. I live to please everyone so I won't be wrecked and ruined. I lose every fight. Poor me, I always get hurt when I try to stand up for myself. I need peace and quiet and should keep my mouth shut, whether people do good or bad.

"It's worthwhile to deceive and to lie instead of always telling the truth. It's better to acquire than to lose, better to run away from the mighty than to obstruct their way. Let them laugh at me—I know what I have and like my little home, my castle. You risk everything if you tell the truth. The fighter dies in the fight" (LVM).

Healing Words of God's Victory

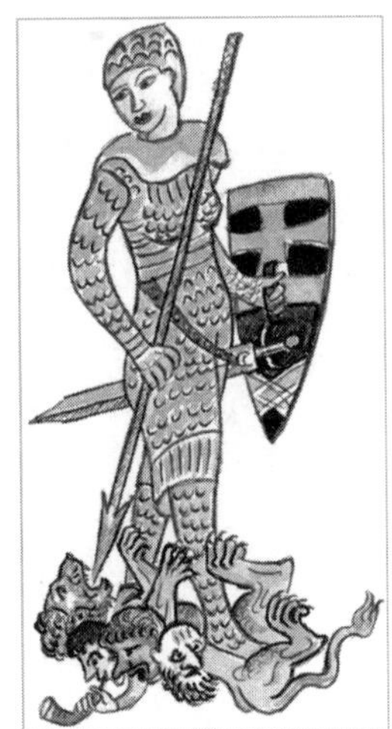

People afflicted with cowardice must learn to trust in God in order to compensate for their negative emotions. The powerful God's Victory rejoices:

"Since the beginning you spoke against God, and you are greatly in error when you give up justice. . . . Therefore, you live with fear and trembling in exile, because you deceive people.

"I am the sword of all virtues and the slayer of all injustice. You will have my sword in your jaw if you are cowardly. Pitiless, I will fight against you, ashes to ashes. Your objectives are too inferior, meaningless, and small. I hate a senseless life in vanity.

"I like to enjoy the full life and the source of life's energy. I kill the old dragon and 'take the helmet of salvation, and the sword of the Spirit, which is the word of God' (Ephesians 6:17)" (LVM).

Cowardice is a virus. It kills the power of the immune system. Whenever we feel down, stressed, and resigned, our immune systems breaks down and diseases go from bad to worse. The cry "Nobody can help me" blocks the healing forces in the body. Hope or the feeling of being in God's hands does quite the opposite. Therefore, fight against Cowardice because:

> I conquer the devil and you, oh hatred and jealousy, and you, oh filthiness, together with those playing with false deception. (SC III, vision 3:5)

Organ Relationship

Cowardice, resignation, frustration, and despair are related to the pathology of the nervous system in the cervical region of the vertebrae, especially C5. The nervous system of this region is responsible for skin diseases. The wounded souls of these patients are visible on the skin. Unfortunately, most skin diseases—for example, neurodermitis, acne, and psoriasis—are highly persistent, with a lifelong physical nature that often turns into hay fever or asthma. The frustrated skin patient has usually traveled from doctor to doctor without success and finally gives up in resignation.

Hildegard observes in her vision fiery storms and turbulence, symbols of the suffering of skin-plagued patients:

> I saw black fog, wild storms causing violent thunderstorms, and an immense black fire. (LVM)

Meditation on Cowardice and God's Victory

Cowardice, desperation, and resignation are related to incurability, especially incurability of skin diseases including neurodermitis, psoriasis, and eczema. But there is always hope for a cure with Hildegard's remedies. They heal the skin from inside out. First an analysis of the microflora of the intestines is made. Then the leaky gut is identified. As soon as the gut heals and the microflora are normal, skin diseases can heal.

The skin is the projection screen for the innermost invisible personality. The skin reflects—for everybody who can read it—feelings and emotions, thought and behavior, and even the condition of the digestion and hormone levels. We become red with shame, white with anger, pale from shock, and green before throwing up. We can see if somebody is eating healthy food or fast food or the four kitchen poisons (strawberries, peaches, plums, and leeks) that cause food allergies, depression, and immune weakness.

Almost every skin disease has a psychological cause—the skin is the mirror of the soul. If we don't consider this fact, skin diseases become incurable. Current medicine, for example, treats skin diseases almost entirely from the outside with cortisone creams and lotions or an antibiotic salve. Cortisone and chemicals do not cure, however, but instead damage and destroy, particularly the intestinal microflora, which are responsible for the well-being of the skin. The relationship between the outside skin and the inside mucous membrane of the intestinal tract is greatly neglected, thus causing incurability and resignation. Skin patients run from one dermatologist to the next and the next, all of whom usually treat the skin only from the outside. Finally, the patient gives up.

Spiritual Healing

A helpful therapy is fasting with soup, fennel tea, or hot water for at least a week, using the sauna with brush massage, and wearing scratchy underclothes. It is also very important to practice compassion with other people according to the instructions of the fasting master.

With the words of Psalms 21 and 45, I Corinthians 15:54–58, and I John 5:1–5, the cowardly person can practice regaining God's victory!

6.	***Ira***	***Patientia***
	Anger	**Tranquillity**
	Impatience	Patience
	Fury	Gentleness
	Rage	Composure
	Aggression	Kindness
	Madness	Peacefulness
	Criminality	Serenity

Crystal Therapy

You'll need a chalcedony bracelet, necklace, or flat stone.

Place it on the artery of the neck or wrist to combat stress, anger, and impatience.

The gold cure is a universal prophylactic and therapeutic remedy for immune modulation: The weak immune system becomes stimulated; the autoaggressive immune system changes to normal. Writes Hildegard: "The gold cure works such that the healthy person stays healthy and the sick patient gets healthy." Hildegard's gold cure is an effective remedy against all autoaggressive sicknesses, like cancer, polyarthritis, fibromyalgia, and even AIDS. The gold cure helps prevent flu and other illnesses caused by colds, which can create complications in elderly people. The fine gold dust does not dissolve and is nontoxic. It strengthens the immune system over the mucous lining of the intestines, where the greatest part of the immune system is located.

Good as Gold

The gold cure is nontoxic and stays in the intestines for about 2 months.

1.2 grams gold powder from a natural source (gold nugget or river gold)
2 tablespoons whole white spelt flour mixed with water into a paste

Stir the gold powder into the paste and divide the mixture into 2 parts. On the first day, eat half the gold paste 30 minutes before breakfast.

Bake the second half into a gold cookie and eat this on the second day.

Note: Repeat once a year.

According to Hildegard of Bingen, the origins of evil are to be found in anger and impatience. War, crime, horror, atrocity, and all the other wickedness of the world are a result of malignancy, which is a part of our human nature. There is no personal without it, and nobody can destroy the evil of the world. All the attempts to demolish evil have created more evil. Human history is an illustrated example of the war against evil: the Crusades, the Inquisition, atomic bombs, high-tech weapons, Desert Storm, and antiterrorism in Afghanistan have not been able to eliminate evil—because evil is a part of life.

Evil originates from a biochemical chain reaction that begins when we become angry. Black bile or gallic acid, a steroid substance related to the sex hormones, is produced in the liver and acidifies the blood and intestines. We become acidic, which causes inflammation, and this leads to autoaggression—our own immune systems rebel against our own bodies. There is no organ, no tissue, no part of the body that cannot be destroyed by autoaggression, a symbol of suicide.

Many of the really bothersome diseases of today, such as cancer, stroke, heart attack, gastritis, colitis, hepatitis, arthritis, and even polyarthritis, result from anger or impatience caused by the black bile boiling up.

Management of anger is the greatest challenge for humanity, because anger destroys not only our own bodies but also life itself.

With its claws and snake feet Anger is pictured in a mill wheel spitting fire and destruction. The head looks like a human skull but has a scorpion mouth. The hands are crippled, with long claws. The body looks like that of a crayfish but with snakes for legs. Hands and feet are stuck in the wheel. Anger is naked and bald, and fire is coming out of his mouth.

Harmful Words of Anger

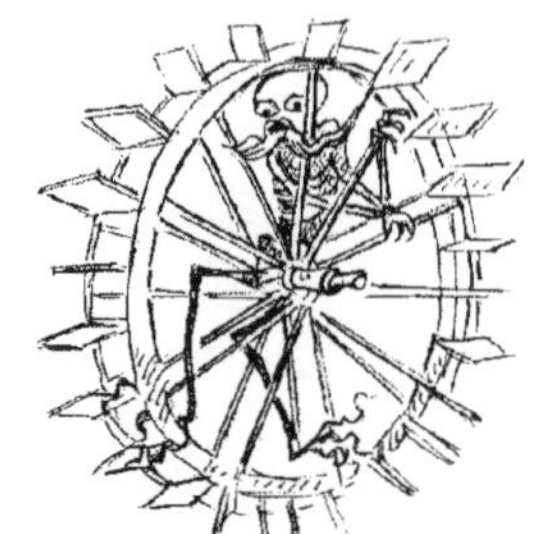

Anger speaks:

"I crush and destroy everything that gets in my way. . . . Why should I permit unfairness? If you like serenity, leave me alone. If anyone wants to hurt me, I will hit him with a sword and break everything to pieces with a club" (LVM).

Nothing can stop us from blowing up when somebody gets in our way except to achieve tranquillity.

Healing Words of Tranquillity

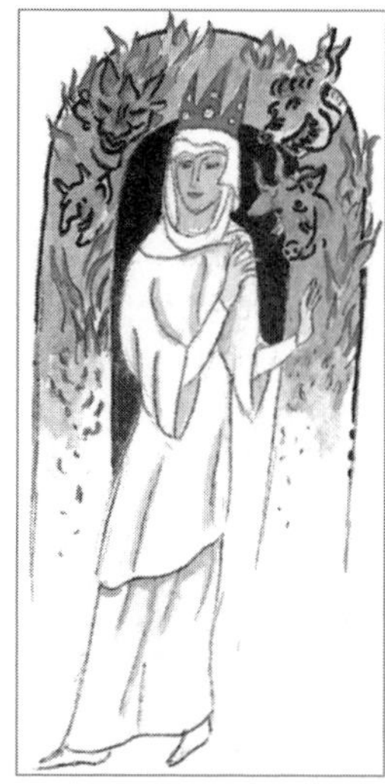

Tranquillity replies:

"My voice echoes over the highest mountains and extends beyond the world. I exude serenity like meditation balm out of the earth. You, however, are the parasite, the bloodsucker, and crime itself.

"I am the sweet life energy, *viriditas.* I bear the flowers and fruits of all virtues and give the heart and spirit strength and energy against destruction. I bring everything I start to a good end. I am aware of evil and handle Anger with gentle tranquillity.

"I destroy no one! I try to live in harmony with everyone. Nobody hates me. But I will destroy your anger, because I remain forever" (LVM).

Practice Patience

Patience can be a big help against anger. Before you blow up, celebrate a ritual.

- Remember the word of God, as in Psalms 23, 91, and 103.
- Make yourself a glass of quenched wine (see page 241) and drink it with your enemy until he becomes your friend.
- Wear a blue chalcedony around your neck or on your wrist to neutralize black bile and help against stress.
- Always look for the sense behind the nonsense and the message or answer to a question like: What is life teaching me right now?
- Compare the attack with the consequences. Good creates good; evil creates evil.
- Be realistic—there will always be injustice. Take the sting out of wickedness by laughing at it.
- Compare your own misery with the injustice that happened to Jesus.

Patience is the best and cheapest tranquilizer. It calms anger and comforts a person. Hildegard writes:

> I conquer in the beginning with the strong Son of God. He came from God for the redemption of people, and he returned to God. He died on the cross with the greatest suffering. But he has risen from the dead and returned to heaven. In the remembrance of this fact, I do not flee from the miseries and the sorrows of this life. (SC III, vision 3)

THE LESSONS OF TRANQUILLITY

Here are the spiritual means to overcome anger and impatience. The application of Hildegard's psychotherapeutic methods could revolutionize the incompetent rehabilitation system of today. Convicts would have a chance for real healing and to learn how to manage their anger. This would be a way out of violence and an opportunity to produce peace in society, and save a lot of money.

1. Inherited anger with permanent odiousness: Practice severe fasting, wear scratchy clothes, apply a brush massage, and sweat in the sauna.
2. Occasional sudden anger without hate: Practice normal fasting, wear scratchy clothes, apply a brush massage, and sweat in the sauna.
3. Murder caused by anger: Practice severe, long-lasting fasting, apply a hard brush massage, withdraw into darkness, get guidance from a fasting master.
4. Murder in greed and avarice: Practice severe, long-lasting fasting, apply a hard brush massage, go into isolation in the loneliness of nature.
5. Justifiable homicide (in self-defense): Practice normal fasting.
6. Unintentional murder out of ignorance, professional error during an operation: Practice normal fasting.
7. Murder by poison or strangulation: Practice severe long-lasting fasting, apply a hard brush massage, wear scratchy clothes, and live like a hermit alone in nature.
8. Abortion, murder of children: Practice severe fasting, apply hard brush massage, wear scratchy clothes, live in isolation in nature.
9. Suicide: Self-punishment is impossible.

Repentance and spiritual healing occur only voluntarily and can never be forced on someone. It is important to know that God does not destroy anybody. Even the murderer has his chance. Remember, the murderer Saint Dismas, who died on the cross with Jesus, was the first man promised paradise and he became a saint.

WHY WE BECOME SICK AND AUTOAGGRESSIVE: THE SILENT SUICIDE

In countless practices today Mr. or Ms. Patient hears the following: "You have cancer [or polyarthitis or neurodermitis] and according to conventional medicine, this is an incurable disease. We do not know the cause and have no cure. You just have to accept life's circumstances. But we can help you handle the symptoms with conventional medical methods like surgery, radiation, and chemotherapy."

This is, in principle, the standard answer for patients with so-called incurable diseases. In 80 percent of all cases, the diseases have two main origins: lifestyle and nutrition. Diseases will always be incurable if these two causes are neglected.

Most of today's sicknesses can be traced to an autoaggressive origin, which means the body destroys itself. Hildegard traces the cause of autoaggression to a chemical substance that she calls black bile, gallic acid, or in Latin *melancholia*. This substance, like cortisone, is released under stress from the liver and quickly discharged into the intestines, which become so acidic that the good bacteria die. Unfortunately, the microflora are the first line of defense against aggressors from the outside.

Leaky-gut Syndrome

Under normal conditions, the acidity of the blood is neutral and the pH is 7.4. With too much black bile the blood becomes acidic and the whole body can become inflamed. The intestinal microflora also suffer under the acidity and destroy the bacteria that usually protect the gut. From now on the contents of the gut can penetrate the blood, causing autointoxicaton. The contents of the gut contain infectious material of bacterial, viral, and protozoan origin as well as a great deal of toxic and allergenic material.

The cost of detoxification is very high. The liver, through which all substances must pass before entering the blood for transport to other organs, and the immune system are both alarmed. Each produces an armada of sophisticated weapons against the intruders—more than one hundred different weapons such as killer cells, free radicals, enzymes, poisonous substances, and other phagocytosic cells that kill the enemies. If the invasion through the mucous leak continues, the immune system produces so many weapons that they enter the bloodstream and destroy body tissue and organs, which become inflamed from the increased acidity. Every cell can be attacked by the autoaggressive immune system.

The leaky gut is the key to understanding the pathogenesis of all inflammatory diseases, including cancer. Free radicals especially are very aggressive; they can penetrate into the cellular genetic material and destroy the genes that are responsible for cellular growth during reproduction. As soon as the little watchdog that looks after the size of a cell dies, the next cell grows uncontrolled and becomes carcinogenic. In a short time we have two, then four, sixteen, two hundred fifty-six cells. It takes years, depending on the type of cancer, until a tumor reaches the size of a pea and is detectable. At this stage there are already billions of cancer cells, yet only now does the treatment begin with surgery, chemotherapy, and radiation. It is much too late, because the tumor is already there and the precious time in the precancer stage has been lost. If the tumor is removed and no change in lifestyle and nutrition occurs, it will return with many more daughter cells.

In cases of stroke and heart attack, the weapons of the immune system inflame and destroy the tissue of the blood vessels, and the resulting vasculitis ruptures vessels in the brain or heart. More than 20,000 different diseases find their origin in bitterness, which Hildegard described 850 years ago in her visionary medical book *Causae et Curae.*

When the human soul feels angry, disagreeable, or irritable, the heart, liver, and blood vessels contract. At the same time a nebula (composed of free radicals) arises and darkens the heart, so the person becomes melancholic. Melancholy produces sadness and bitterness. As soon as we notice depression, the nebula, which shrouded the heart in darkness, heats up a hot gas in all humors and produces bile. The acid of the bile causes more anger.

The bile disappears when the person is able to cope with the situation (through spirituality, prayer, meditation, or another antistress measure). If the situation does not change, the gases excite the black bile and produce a very black nebula, and the liver produces even more acidity. The gases move up to the head and destroy the brain, then descend and penetrate the stomach to damage the intestines (leaky-gut syndrome) and cause other sicknesses (such as dementia).

Many other severe diseases develop from the acidic humors of bile and black bile. "Man would always be healthy if he didn't have the acidity of black bile" (CC, 146:4).

Autoaggression and Black Bile

The following diseases are the result of autoaggression due to black bile:

- Allergy, hay fever, eczema, acne, psoriasis, asthma
- Cancer
- Chronic fatigue syndrome
- Chronic inflammatory arthritis
- Fibromyalgia, scleroderma, lupus erythematosus
- Gastritis, colitis, Crohn's disease, celiac disease, hepatitis, pancreatitis, nephritis
- Heart attack
- Migraine, depression, Alzheimer's disease, Parkinson's disease, multiple sclerosis
- Stroke

Effective treatment of leaky-gut syndrome requires several steps in order to change lifestyle. Spiritual healing is necessary, and there are appropriate strategies to reverse the intestinal permeability and to neutralize black bile.

THE CHAOS OF THE DEFENSE SYSTEM: MICROBACTERIAL DYSBACTERIA

One hundred trillion microorganisms—ten times more than the total of our body cells—live in our intestines in just two hundred square meters, about half the size of a football field. The microflora are of great importance and provide us with all the nutrients we need: proteins, carbohydrates, fat, minerals, and trace minerals. The normal gut microflora are also capable of synthesizing all vitamins. But many external and internal poisons destroy the bacterial gut flora, resulting in malnutrition and a deficiency of essential nutrients, including vitamins and minerals. This is why so many Americans think they have to take megadoses of industrially made supplements.

Dysbacteria can cause bacterial overgrowth with pathogenic organisms like severe candida infections. Among other problems, these infections create gut inflammation and injury to the intestinal wall. The proper functioning of the intestinal microflora is carelessly neglected by conventional medicine. Yogurt with artificial probiotics from the food industry causes even greater damage.

DAMAGE OF THE GUT MICROFLORA BY MEDICINE

Many medications taken by mouth destroy the normal microflora, especially antibiotics, cortisone, hormone pills, and anti-inflammatory drugs like aspirin and indomethacin. The constant use of painkillers for arthritis damages the lining of the stomach and intestines by inhibiting the synthesis of protective prostaglandins and can result in gastritis and ulcers. After antibiotic therapy, the intestinal mucous lining looks as cratered as the surface of the moon and cries for repair.

From this point of view, it is crystal clear that the resulting ailments from autoaggression will stay incurable as long as the microflora are not repaired.

PRACTICAL APPROACHES TO CURE AUTOAGGRESSION

The first step in breaking the vicious cycle is an analysis of the gut flora by a good microbiological institute. The practical screening test of the microflora shows the degree of the leaky-gut syndrome and the status of the immune system. The test includes the status of the microflora of the upper small intestine and the colon as well as the presence of pathogenic yeast, *Helicobacter pylori,* and other infectious bacterial, viral, or protozoan and parasitic pathogens. The presence of leukocytes is a sign of intestinal inflammation and the degree of the intestinal permeability.

Intestinal permeability can also be tested by the amount of lactulose/mannitol excretion. This test was proposed for the first time by Claude André at l'Hôpital St. Vincent de Paul in Paris for the detection of food allergies. In the Hildegard practice we measure permeability with the indican excretion test. Indican is a substance normally excreted from the colon and found in urine only if the gut is leaky.

Dysbiosis and intestinal permeability require immediate measures. Historically, intestinal purgation was one of the most important healing procedures. The famous medieval physician Paracelsus, who died in 1541 in Salzburg, recommended colon cleansing, because he believed death began in the intestinal tract *(Der Tod sitzt im Darm).*

This is the optimal mixture, more precious than gold and more useful than pure gold. With its help migraine disappears. It cleanses the damp lung, which is caused by eating raw pears, and consumes all bad humors (mali humores) that are in humans.

Pear Honey

A few years ago I discovered that Hildegard's remedy Anthamanticum with pear honey (Mel piratum) *is a powerful cleansing and healing mixture in the fight against intestinal pathogens, including candida.*

8 pears, cored and seeded
35 grams bear fennel rhizome (Radix anthamanticum)
28 grams little galangal rhizome (Radix galangal minor)
22 grams licorice rhizome (Radix liquiritiae)
15 grams summer savory (Satureja hortensis)
8 tablespoons defoamed honey (put honey in a glass in a pan of boiling water, stir, and remove foam)

Cut the pears into small pieces and simmer enough water to cover until the pears are soft.

Strain, then beat until you have a sauce.

Mix the fennel, galangal, licorice, and summer savory to form a powder. Blend into the pear pulp. Add the honey and stir until the mixture is the consistency of jam.

Spoon into a jar, cover, and refrigerate.

Take 1 teaspoon in the morning, 2 teaspoons at lunch, and 3 teaspoons before bedtime, either straight from the spoon or spread on a piece of bread.

Note: Children and sensitive people should cut each amount in half.

In addition, take natural acidophilus/bifidus probiotics, and if necessary *E. coli* (sold as Mutafor) or other missing bacteria for the regeneration of the microflora. Investigate the result four weeks after the intestinal cleansing.

DIETARY MEASURES: SPELT, VEGETABLES, AND FRUITS

Vegetables, grains (especially the oldest grain, spelt), and fruits contain all the minerals and trace minerals necessary for the regeneration of bones, ligaments, tissues, and membranes. At the same time, minerals are alkaline and neutralize gallic and uric acid, thereby fighting inflammation. Animal protein in meat, cheese, eggs, and milk products should be reduced, as it is metabolized to uric acid, which again causes inflammation.

Many red and yellow vegetables and fruits contain bioflavonoids, which are potent antioxidants that fight against free radicals. They all block allergic and autoaggressive reaction. Most important are:

- Pumpkins, beets, carrots, cherries, black and red currants, blackberries.
- Dietary supplements with highly soluble fiber sources, such as fruit pectin in apples and psyllium (fleawort seeds), which reverse the permeability of the intestines by forming a protective film over the inflamed wall and stimulating mucous growth factors. Low-insoluble fibers as in wheat bran increase permeability.
- Duckweed elixir, a complex mixture of several herbs that modulates the aggressive immune system and is effective in eliminating immune impairment and stopping inflammation.

Organ Relationship

Anger and impatience not only lead to aggression and crime but also lower the interferon level and weaken the immune system. They are related to the pathology of the nervous system in the cervical region of the vertebrae, especially C6. The nervous system here is responsible for the gastrointestinal system. The results of anger and impatience become visible in the autoaggression illnesses of our time, just as with cancer a visible lump is a sign of an invisible problem. The sickness usually starts in the gastrointestinal system as gastritis, colitis, or leaky-gut syndrome.

There is always hope for a cure with Hildegard's remedies and with the search to heal the disease by finding its cause and origin. We can discover autoaggression through an analysis of the microflora and by looking for leucocytes in the feces, which reveal inflammation and a leaky gut. As soon as the gut heals and the microflora are normalized, autoaggression has no point anymore from which to destroy the body.

Spiritual Healing

All crimes are an outcome of anger. It is only anger in the consciousness that makes crime happen. Sometimes propaganda can make a whole nation angry, so that the people go astray and become aggressive and evil. Learn to practice patience.

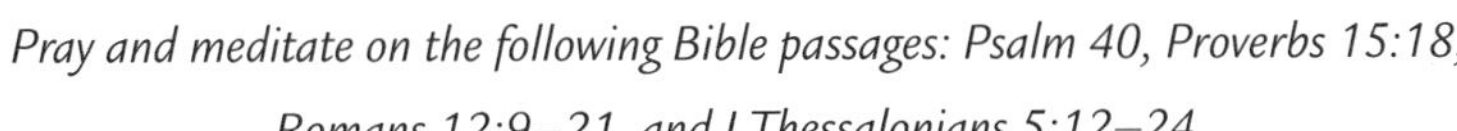
Pray and meditate on the following Bible passages: Psalm 40, Proverbs 15:18, Romans 12:9–21, and I Thessalonians 5:12–24.

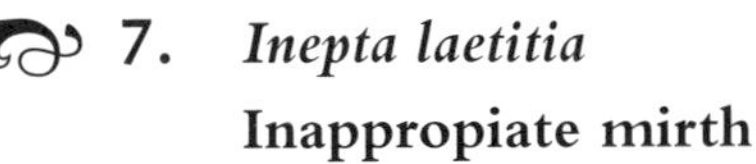

7.	***Inepta laetitia***	***Gemitus ad Deum***
	Inappropiate mirth	**Yearning for God**
	Making fun of someone	Looking for the good
	Cynicism	Cheerfulness
	Satire, mockery	Longing for paradise
	Malicious joy	Good humor

Crystal Therapy

Two crystal therapies apply.

Rock crystal water. Cut a piece of quartz into a small disk and place it in direct sunlight until it is hot. Deposit the hot quartz in a pitcher of fresh water, and drink the water or use it for everything you drink or cook. The rock crystal water cleanses the thyroid gland and is helpful for hormone regulation to prevent goiter in cases of hyper- or hypofunction of the thyroid gland.

Onyx wine. Place an onyx in a glass of wine and leave overnight. Then boil the wine, with the stone it it, for 5 minutes. Remove the stone and drink the wine. Or use the wine to make a spelt soup (see below). This helps swollen lymph glands and a swollen spleen.

Creamed Spelt Soup

1/2 cup butter
1/4 cup spelt flour
5 cups water or vegetable stock
herbs, salt, and pepper to taste

Melt butter in a 2-quart saucepan over medium heat. Add spelt flour and cook, stirring constantly with a wooden spoon, for about 3 minutes or until the flour browns. Add water or vegetable stock to saucepan and beat until smooth. Reduce the heat to low, and add herbs, salt, and pepper. Allow mixture to simmer uncovered for 30 minutes, stirring occasionally. Do not boil.

We are strangers on earth. The human soul lives as an alien in her house with an indelible but vague memory of her divine home. We live here in this distressed world with the permanent knowledge that this place could be enjoyable, but it is not. There is usually someone who likes trouble. His problem is inappropriate mirth—the opposite of brightness or joy in God. On the other hand, some people live on the sunny side of life with an innate good humor and bring sunshine and well-being wherever they go.

Inappropriate Mirth looks like a satyr—a man with monkey hands and goat legs—and his roar of laughter injures the spleen. In contrast to Good Humor or the high spirit of cheerfulness, cynicism is toxic and hurts like the guffaw tactlessly blurted out by Mr. Mockery.

Harmful Words of Inappropriate Mirth

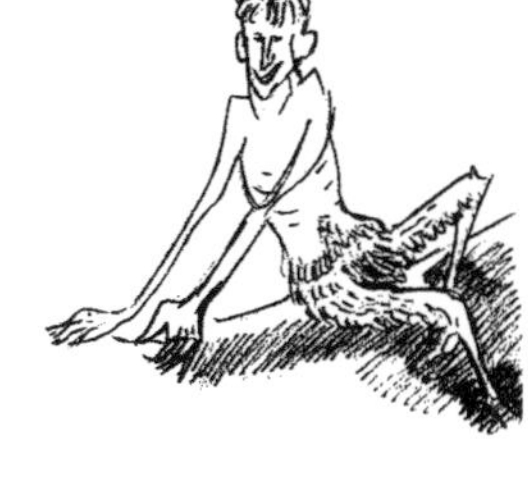

Inappropriate Mirth speaks:

"I am the sweet life! La dolce vita is beautiful. Why should I live in abstinence? God created me and gave me this life. Shall I not live for the pleasures of my beautiful body? Why should I kill my nature? I know the lust of this world and will live according to my desire and enjoy life in excess" (LVM).

Sighing to God is the sound of repentance heard as a voice from a storm cloud.

Healing Words of Yearning for God

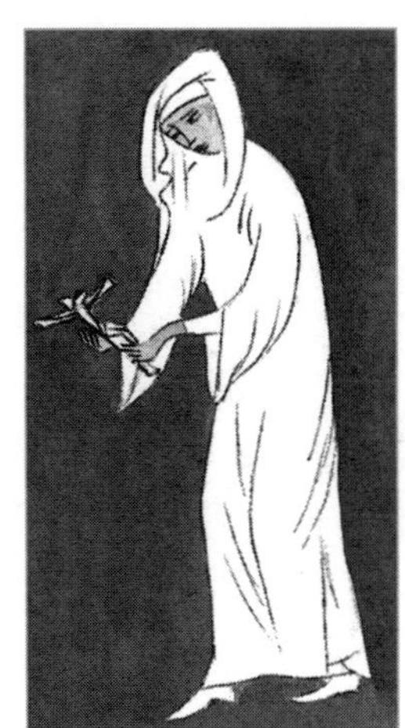

Yearning for God speaks:

"You naked monster, why aren't you red with shame? Your life is no more than obscurity and a shadow of the night. Your behavior ignores all the limits of justice and honesty. You don't live a reasonable life—it is rather chaotic, destructive, and harmful. But I know very well that all earthly life withers like grass into hay. Therefore, I long for another existence that will never end. I am searching for celestial harmony and heavenly joy. I live in the company of angels and enjoy spiritual gifts. That is my real life and that is where I belong" (LVM).

Organ Relationship

The targets of inappropriate mirth, cynicism, malicious joy, and mockery cure the spleen, the lymphatic system, and vertebra C7, the last in the cervical region. The spleen is the filter organ to cleanse dead blood cells. It is the "grave of the leukocytes." The spleen is also responsible for the metabolism of the heart. The spleen suffers and swells from rough food and kitchen poisons like leeks, strawberries, peaches, and plums, which cause black bile, allergy, and inflammation. Hildegard's heart wine (below) cleanses the spleen of its poisons and takes away heart pain.

Hildegard's parsley-honeywine is a delicious and effective remedy and it is easy to make. This ideal combination of heart medicine and heart tonic does relieve pains in the heart, spleen, and side.

Take 8 to 10 parsley leaves with stems. Boil in 1 quart of natural red or white wine with 2 tablespoons wine vinegar for 5 minutes. Add 3/4 cup honey (1/3 cup or less for diabetics) and heat up again for 5 minutes. Skim off the foam, strain, and rebottle the wine.

Take 1 to 5 tablespoons daily and all gripping, shooting heart pain, caused by weather or excitement, will disappear. You don't have to be afraid—heart wine can never harm you. Not only the initial light heart pain disappears, but even severe heart pain caused by chronic rheumatic disease or by heart insufficiency can be healed. Parsley-honeywine is valuable in cases of rehabilitation after heart attacks, too. It does not matter whether you use red or white wine, but it should be a natural wine, without additives.

Spiritual Healing

Spiritual healing occurs during fasting and leads to real joy and a desire for God.

The first three days of fasting are dramatic as the body gets rid of its wastes. Once this is accomplished, the fasting person enters a stage of enlightenment, happiness, satisfaction, and even ecstasy, such that the world becomes a wonderful place.

The Desire for God is present in the words of Psalms 73, 142, and 143 and in I Corinthians 14:1–3 and Colossians 4:2–6.

Chapter 4

The Westman

Hildegard observes the cosmic man turning west and recognizes the second group of virtues and vices from his shoulders to his hips. In this section are the virtues and vices from eight to fifteen, which are related to the psychological risk factors of the intestinal tract. The Westman symbolizes the torso from the shoulders to the lower limbs, which contains the gastrointestinal tract and the lungs, heart, liver, pancreas, and kidneys. This area is especially innervated from the autonomic nervous center and is related to the thoracic bones 1–8, responsible for the functioning and health of the stomach and intestines.

The virtues of this group are healing forces for gastrointestinal diseases. The vices can cause sickness in the same region. The strength of the autonomic nervous system is a result of a healthy pregnancy. A pregnancy under severe pressure can cause a predisposition for disease in this area. Some people who as babies had too much strain during gestation will swallow trouble and sadness later in life and be unable to digest them. This can cause gastritis, diarrhea, or constipation due to damage to the intestinal microflora.

The second group of eight virtues and vices is important for the development of a healthy child during pregnancy. Any transgression might have a harmful influence on the baby and his later life. Chronic inflammation like gastritis, gastric ulcer, stomach or colon cancer, colitis, Crohn's disease, and sprue (celiac disease) can be the result of the eight risk factors during pregnancy.

8.	*Ingluvies ventri* (gluttony)	*Abstinentia* (abstinence)
9.	*Acerbitas* (bitterness of heart)	*Vera largitas* (generosity)
10.	*Impietas* (wickedness)	*Pietas* (devotion)
11.	*Fallacitas* (lying)	*Veritas* (truth)
12.	*Contentio* (contention, war)	*Pax* (peace)
13.	*Infelicitas* (unhappiness)	*Beatitudo* (blessedness)
14.	*Immoderatio* (immoderation)	*Discretio* (discretion)
15.	*Perditio animarum* (lost soul)	*Salvatio animarum* (saved soul)

8. ***Ingluvies ventri*** / ***Abstinentia***

Gluttony	**Abstinence**
Overeating	Eating in moderation
Indulgence	Sobriety

Crystal Therapy

The diamond is an appetite suppressant.

Have a diamond set in gold hanging on a chain for frequent use. To suppress appetite, lick the diamond. This is practical for use during fasting.

All evil in mankind started with a forbidden meal from the tree of the knowledge of good and evil. From that time on humankind wished to be like God and thought it could exterminate evil. But all attempts to eradicate evil failed—in fact, evil became worse than before.

Hildegard writes about evil often and in great detail. Evil is there even as a part of human nature. The art of a meaningful life results from the balance between good and evil without any attempt to be "like God."

The first pair in this section illustrate gluttony and abstinence. The glutton worships its belly and eats itself to death. The form Gluttony looks like a snake rolling on its back, a symbol of an upset gastrointestinal tract. Her eyes glow like fire and her tongue sticks out. Her belly is transparent.

Harmful Words of Gluttony

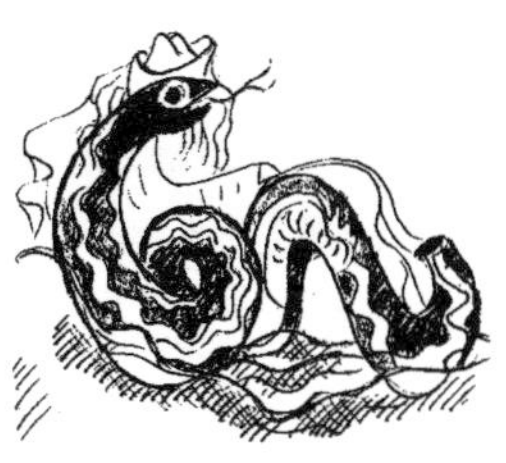

Gluttony speaks:

"God has created everything; why should I renounce anything? If God had not known we need all this, he would not have made it. I would be crazy not to pamper my appetite" (LVM).

Abstinence is a protection not only from overeating but also from the damage of too much alcohol, overindulgence or intoxication with drugs, nicotine, or even too much sex, especially during pregnancy. The people in the West suffer not from starvation but instead from overeating and overindulgence in every respect. Gluttony causes civilization illnesses like stroke, heart attack, and cancer.

Healing Words of Abstinence

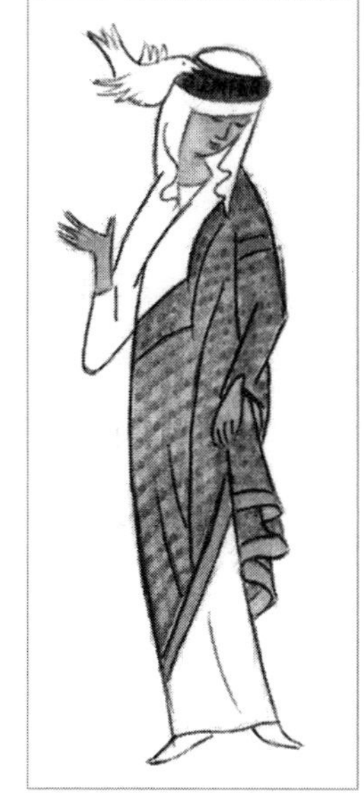

Abstinence responds:

"Nobody plays the harp by ripping the strings to pieces. You, Gluttony, stuff your belly until your veins burst and you are doubled over with cramps. Where is the wisdom you received from God? The excesses from meat and wine ruin the body just as sudden heavy rains flood the earth.

"I esteem the beautiful image of man and woman made of clay. I take care and respect human nature and eat and drink in moderation. I vibrate in beautiful harmony like a harp when I eat with discretion. The entire universe resounds with me like an organ.

"You, Gluttony, have no understanding, because sometimes you fast like a madman and other times you eat until you burst.

"I eat in moderation, enjoying myself and delighting in my body, which generates good humors and acquires a good disposition. I sing with the organ and pray with the harp. This keeps me away from gluttony and the obsession with my belly" (LVM).

Abstinence, like fasting, is a simple way to change our lifestyles and transform our behavior. In refusing to eat to excess, we save digestive energy and gain uplifting life energy. Abstinence renounces not only food but also wealth out of love of God. Blessed is the child of the mother who knows the secrets of the spirit of sacrifice. Abstinence compensates for gluttony and restores balance.

The pregnant mother should, therefore, consider Hildegard's advice for food and how to eat it, because food is the medicine most important for the health of her baby. She should also live in accordance with the healing powers of the virtues and in so doing influence the character of the child while still in the womb.

> I am filled with inner mercy, from which little rivulets spring forth. I do not wish to conceal any wealth, gold, precious stones, or pearls from needy people and from those suffering lack who are lamenting. I will comfort them now and will relieve their poverty on account of my love for the Word of God, which is sweet and soft and which passes out good things to their souls. The Word touches the wounds of their sins because of their repentance. (Wisdom 11:23) (SC III, vision 6:1)

Gluttony is the mother of all obsessions including work, alcohol, drugs, medicines, birth-control pills, nicotine, and sex. All obsessions and their sister, Gluttony, are constantly looking for the lost paradise or its substitute. The belly becomes God as seen in every gourmet restaurant.

"But the kingdom of God is not only eating and drinking."

—ROMANS 14:17

FOODS THAT CREATE ACID

Too much food—especially animal foods like meat, cheese, and eggs—makes us heavy and earthy. Animal food produces acid by increasing not only the uric acid but also melancholy, known scientifically as gallic acid. Melancholy is biochemically related to the steroid cholesterol, a precursor of the sex hormones. It has been shown that an excess of sex hormones causes cancers of the breast, colon, and prostate. In addition, animal protein acidifies the blood, all the organs, and all the tissues, causing inflammation and autoaggression.

Vegetarians have a natural protection against cancer because their hormones are in balance. Mother Earth's wisdom protects vegetarians not only from the mistakes of the food industry like mad cow disease and many other viral infections but also from getting sour!

Organ Relationship

Gluttony, overeating, and indulgence are related to the pathology of the nervous system in the thoracic-lumbar region of the vertebrae, especially Th1. The nervous system here controls the gastrointestinal area including the digestive organs—the liver, gallbladder, and pancreas. Inflammation and autoaggression in these organs are often caused by gluttony and include sicknesses that end with *itis,* such as gastritis, colitis, hepatitis, and pancreatitis.

Spiritual Healing

Spiritual healing of gluttony, overindulgence, and excess occurs with spiritual food like the divine energy coming from prayer, meditation, and fasting under the authority of a fasting master.

Use the following Bible passages for prayer and study: Romans 14:5–8, I Timothy 3:1–5 and verse 11, Titus 2:1–8, and Peter 2:9–12.

9.	*Acerbitas*	*Vera largitas*
	Bitterness of heart	**Generosity**
	Rudeness	Kindness
	Being sour	Practicing goodwill
	Intolerance	Tolerance
	Fanaticism	Open-mindedness

Crystal Therapy

Chalcedony and sapphire are important aspects of crystal therapy.

Place a chalcedony bracelet, necklace, or flat stone on the artery of the neck or wrist to combat stress, anger, and impatience.

Another help against sudden stress or anger is a sapphire placed in the mouth.

The second negative force is bitterness—the bitterness of black bile, which poisons the blood and acidifies the body. Bitterness is the result of gluttony. Overeating leads to indigestion, decay, and bitterness. Bitterness is no longer human; it looks like a leopard.

Harmful Words of Bitterness of Heart

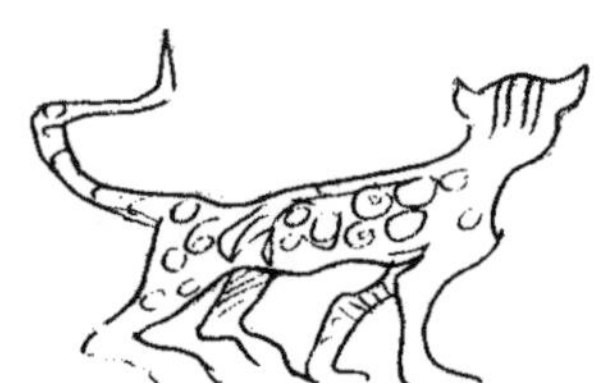

This egoistic vice speaks:

"Courage and victory do not impress me. I don't want anyone to stand in my way. I won't even bother to answer those who annoy me or could harm me with their writing and beliefs. I simply ignore them" (LVM).

Healing Words of Generosity

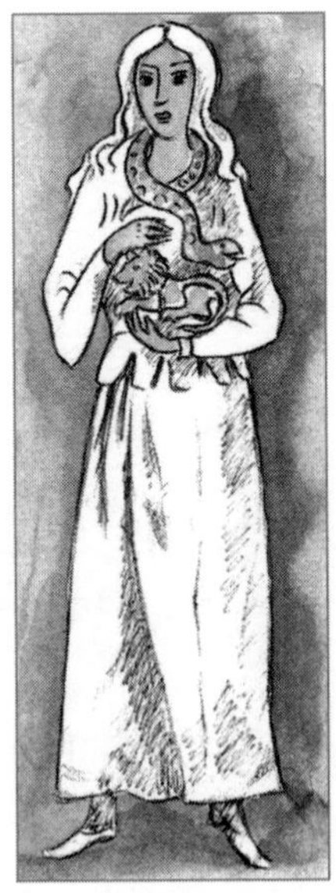

Generosity bases her life on spiritual principles that are sweeter than bitterness. Like rain and dew, salve and medicine, Generosity is open and ready to spread joy, mercy, and comfort:

"You are a very dangerous, evil, injurious, and destructive shadow. You live irresponsibly and in conflict with God and his law. I am open-hearted and spread comfort and encouragement, which are just as effective as medicine or ointment. I am a remedy, full of joy and compassion, ready to fight sickness and tribulation. Nobody can stop me from doing this and I will survive forever. Your origin is death and hell" (LVM).

Generosity looks up to the radiant lion, a symbol for Jesus, which nourishes the poor and the heartbroken out of love of God. If you help the hungry and satisfy the desires of the afflicted, then your light shall rise in the darkness and your sadness will be bright as at noon. Then the Lord will guide you continually and satisfy your desires with good things and make your bones strong.

Generosity is a representative of life and looks to Jesus:

> I look at this bright lion and give an account of his love. But I flee from the burning serpent, and have respect only for the serpent hanging on the tree. (SC, vision 6:2)

THE CHEMISTRY OF BITTERNESS

To function properly, the blood requires stability. The acidity of the blood is indicated by the normal pH of 7.4, which is slightly alkaline. The liver produces extreme amounts of gallic acid when we get angry or eat too much fat. As a result, acidity increases and destroys the environment. Too much gallic acid kills the intestinal microflora, the first line of immune defense. In addition, the increased quantity of gallic acid acidifies the blood, leading to an autoaggressive inflammation of the body's cells and organs. Every cell can be attacked and destroyed.

This harmful acidity is the final cause of all sicknesses. Therefore, it is important to control our thoughts and emotions and thereby control gallic acid in the body. Gallic acids are key members of the important steroids of the body, including sex hormones, the repair hormone cortisone, and the building block of all cell membranes, cholesterol. Too much gallic acid increases the amount of cholesterol and sex hormones and leads to arteriosclerosis and even to tumors of the breast, colon, and prostate.

Organ Relationship

Bitterness of heart, sarcasm, rudeness, and being sour are symbols of aggression sicknesses, which occur after the body becomes acidic. In the pathology of the nervous system, they are related to the vertebra Th2, found in the thoracic-lumbar region of the vertebrae. Acidity is also a visible sign for heartburn and can cause gastritis, ulceration, and cancer of the stomach.

Babies who are born under "acidic conditions" may suffer later from chronic inflammation of the gastrointestinal tract. Even unwanted children, however, can receive the chance of a good life. Mother Teresa saved many babies out of the garbage who later became wonderful human beings.

Hildegard observes in her vision fiery snakes. A snake goes through many generations of skin, a symbol for dry, peeling skin and itching eczema and psoriasis. She writes:

> I saw an immense black fire, full of fiery snakes with burning pale flames coming out of their mouths. The snakes were torturing all the bitter people. They had to suffer and burn because of their infidelity. The pale flame was scorching because of their lust for intolerance. Their bitter character offended the commandments of God, which is why snakes and reptiles tortured them. (LVM)

Meditation on Generosity

Life requires generosity. In particular, the young embryo just conceived is totally dependent on motherly love. The pregnant mother is a natural symbol for generosity; she acts in favor of her baby.

Christmas is the greatest symbol of happiness and joy about a newborn baby. Artists from all countries and all times have overwhelmingly expressed their fascination for Christmas in music, painting, architecture, and poetry. The music of the baroque era was especially rich—listen to Bach's *Christmas Oratorio* and the *Christmas Concertos* of Covelli and Schütz, for example. Close to the Hildegard Kurhaus in Allensbach, in southern Germany, is the baroque jewel on Lake Constance, the church of Birnau. It was built in 1750 by three great baroque artists, who created heaven on earth to reveal generosity in the motherhood of Mary and the baby Jesus, the visible image of the invisible God.

The practice of abortion is an insult against humanity and an insult to the message of Christmas. A real mother will usually become sick, bitter, melancholy, and sour when she is confronted with the idea of abortion. Even the baby physically united with the mother suffers from this bitterness. Later in life a once unwanted baby may suffer from anxiety, problems with digestion, and even thoughts of suicide. An unloved baby is a candidate for suicide and crime. A strong mother resists abortion and develops tremendous joy and energy for her baby and for life.

Spiritual Healing

Spiritual healing of bitterness of heart, sarcasm, and rudeness occurs from spiritual energy regenerated through prayer, meditation, and fasting.

10. *Impietas* / *Pietas*

Wickedness	**Devotion**
Impiety	Piety
Cynicism	Reverence, goodness
Lack of regard for others	High regard, appreciation
Contempt	Respect
Ungodliness	Godliness, veneration

Crystal Therapy

The emerald is helpful for gastro-cardiac pain.

Place an emerald on the skin wherever it hurts.

Gluttony and Bitterness are the parents of Wickedness. Wickedness changes mankind into a monster. The contemptible character has a head like a wild animal projecting out of his chest with fiery eyes and a leopard mouth. Out of the corners of his mouth a snake's head is hanging.

Harmful Words of Wickedness

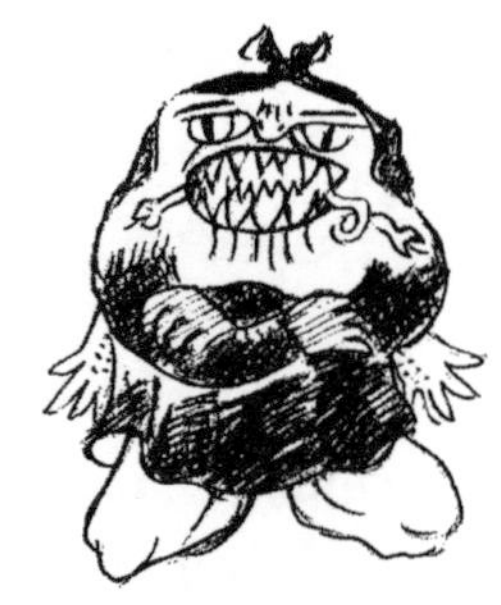

Wickedness speaks:

"I don't want to obey God or any other person. If I listen to anybody else and respect his will, he could take advantage of me and say, 'Do this or do that for me!' I would never allow this. If someone does me wrong, he'll get it back a hundred times. I regulate my own business and nobody should dare to interfere. I will never fall on my knees. Everything I can use I will, just like everyone else does who is not a fool. It doesn't make me feel good to do good just because God wants me to do it" (LVM).

Healing Words of Devotion

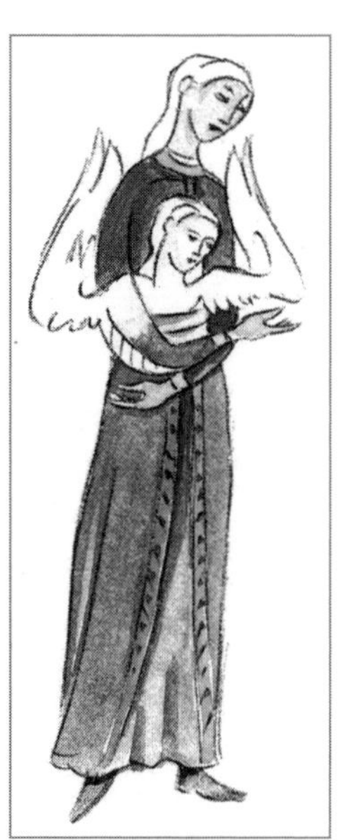

Devotion responds:

"You are devilish, harmful, and malignant. God is not God if he honors your vicious work and rewards your infamy. God throws you into the inferno like a chunk of lead. Where is your power? I see only darkness, heresy, hostility, and destruction. Where do you live? You live where disgrace, insults, and slander rule. Where do you rest? You rest in the confusion and distortion of the truth. Where is your home? Your home is where everybody fights against everybody as in disaster and war. You are never-ending bloodshed" (LVM).

Wickedness needs the positive healing energy of Devotion.
Unbelievers need the help of angels, worship, and adoration in order to get well again. Hildegard writes:

> I have an angel for my companion. I do not want to walk with swindlers who mask themselves, but I do want to celebrate with the just. (SC III, vision 6:3)

Organ Relationship

Wickedness, cynicism, low or no regard for others, and contempt symbolize the pathology of problems connected with the spinal nerves from the thoracic-lumbar region of the vertebrae, especially Th3. The nervous system here controls the gastrointestinal area, including digestive organs like the liver, gallbladder, and the pancreas. In her vision Hildegard describes fire and bubbling blobs of lead mixed with sulfur as symbols for gastritis, ulcers, colitis, and bleeding hemorrhoids, for example:

> I saw a gigantic fire, hot molten lead combined with sulfur. The place was teeming with active worms. All those impetuous people who were occupied with wickedness during their lifetimes had to suffer from these plagues. Worms tortured them because of their fanatic bitterness against their fellow man.

Spiritual Healing

Spiritual healing of wickedness and a lack of reverence is possible during fasting and self-punishment with brush massage under the supervision of a fasting master. It is important that the body play a role in order to learn reverence by kneeling, bowing down, or humbling oneself facedown on a mat.

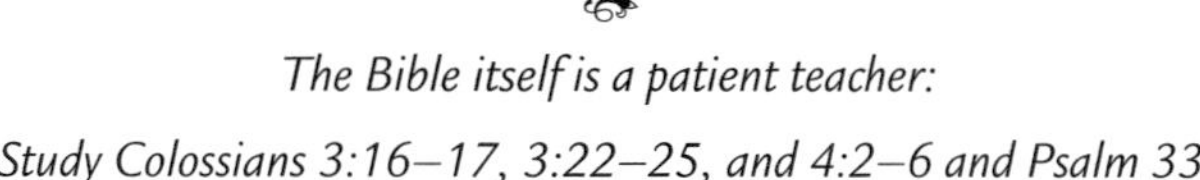

The Bible itself is a patient teacher:

Study Colossians 3:16–17, 3:22–25, and 4:2–6 and Psalm 33.

11. *Fallacitas* — *Veritas*

Lying	**Truth**
Trickery	Integrity
Cheating	Honesty
Falseness	Sincerity
Doubt	Certainty

Crystal Therapy

The diamond is a stress suppressant.

Have a diamond set in gold and hang it on a chain for frequent use. Lick the diamond to suppress fanaticism, lying, and anger.

The next three virtues and vices belong together. Each stimulates the next:

Fallacitas (lying)	*Veritas* (truth)
Contentio (contention)	*Pax* (peace)
Infelicitas (unhappiness)	*Beatitudo* (blessedness)

Lying leads to contention; contention produces unhappiness. Nobody can be happy without peace and truth.

The inclination to lie is common to everyone since the time of paradise. Lying in wait is the "snake-in-the-grass" question:

"Have you ever lied?" Everyone except a liar would answer yes. Only a fool would answer no. The serpent represents the wiggling between the two boundaries of falsehood and truth. We have learned in our lives when it is suitable to lie and when it is better to tell the truth. But we also experience that lying afflicts the good conscience and causes stomachaches. In addition, a pregnancy under extreme pressure can increase the unborn person's inclination to lie.

The wicked go astray from the womb, they err from their birth, speaking lies.

—PSALM 58:3

Harmful Words of Lying

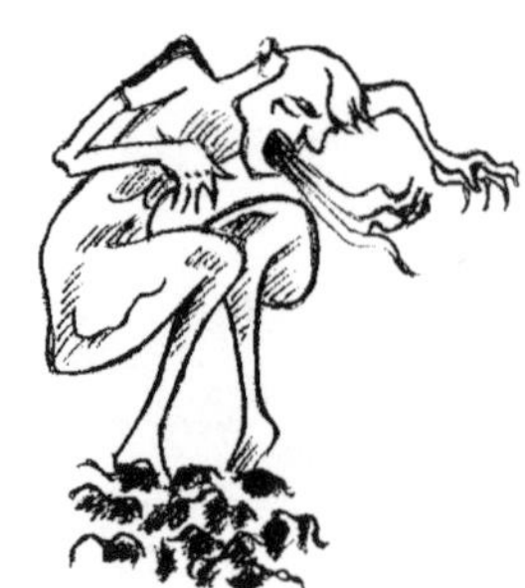

In Hildegard's vision the liar appears surrounded by thick gloomy clouds so that its form is hardly visible. It stands on dry, hard, black foam and expels a scorching flame. The Liar speaks:

"Who can always tell the truth? If I wish my fellow man all the best, I would have to harm myself. It is in my character, a real part of me, to oppress others. I always have new tricks because I never found that someone became distinguished or wealthy without these methods. I want things that I don't have and will do anything, including lying or storytelling, to get them. I would not be wealthy and rich if I always said the truth. My business is lying and cheating in order to receive belongings and property.

"Look at the truth fanatics! They are unpopular, homeless, and possess nothing. I want to be rich and esteemed, more than anyone else is, and show off my wealth. Consequently, I lie and manipulate the truth. I make use of shifting stories to find an advantage. I employ spin doctors to distort the truth in order to bring me even more benefits. This is how all who are rich play the game" (LVM).

Many politicians and diplomats are strong examples of liars who have made it an art to not tell the truth. Diplomats speak French, the language in which everything sounds polite. There is a nice euphemism—they say *corriger la fortune,* which means to manipulate everything in favor of yourself. We also know that some public relations specialists and lawyers play the game of twisting the story. The truth always has two sides, depending on your viewpoint. The American pilots who bombed Vietnam with napalm and Agent Orange were considered war criminals by the North Vietnamese but heroes in South Vietnam and patriots in much of America.

Healing Words of Truth

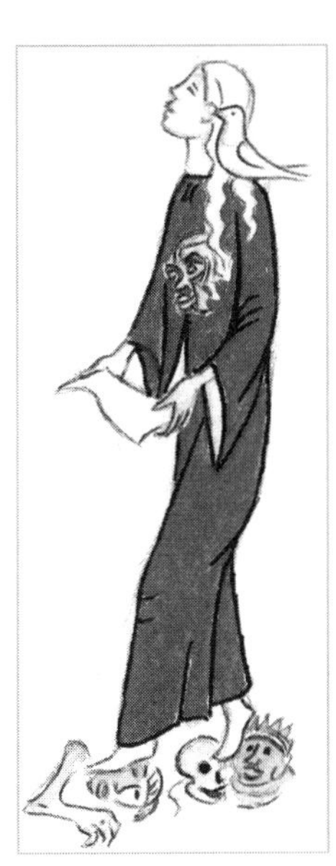

Truth speaks:

"You speak the language of the infernal snake. You stir up the flame of lying and deceit. You are the source of all malignancy. Mendacity flows from your prostitute breasts. You will obtain a reputation as a whore and will lose all your happiness and success.

"I am a landmark who stands strong on the way to God and I sound like the trumpet of almighty justice. I talk about all his admirable works and thereby show the truth. God celebrates his festivities with me in the palace of the king. I am decorated with the splendid jewelry of God and declare the truth of his justice. Heaven and earth and all other creatures, which are the innermost heart of the world, are full of truth. Even the waters that circulate under heaven and earth follow the same truth" (LVM).

If Christ is the truth, then the lie is the Antichrist. The lie has been a powerful instrument to persecute Christians through the centuries.

Truth says in the book *Scivias:*

> I want to be a green stick for the bitter attack to whip the deceitful snake, who is the son of Satan. . . . I contradict and upset the devil. I spit the devil out of my mouth like a deadly poison even though the devil never entered me with his cunning tricks. The devil is the worst of all evils to me because all evil has its source in the devil. Therefore, I throw down the devil and trample him underfoot with the justice of God, who loves me forever. I am a supporter of and a leader for God. All virtues can be built on my foundation, because I am solid and steadfast. (SC III, vision 6:4)

Organ Relationship

Lying and cheating symbolize the pathology of problems connected with the spinal nerves from the thoracic-lumbar region of the vertebrae, especially Th4. The nervous system here controls the gastrointestinal area including the digestive organs—the stomach, colon, liver, gallbladder, and pancreas.

The liar resembles a snake that swallows big chunks at once, like a whole rabbit, without choking. Hildegard writes in her medical book *Causae et Curae* that the stomach mucus becomes green and blue and black as a result of overeating and causes strong pain and gas. Hildegard describes the liar in colorful words:

> I saw a fire burning in the dark and many dragons were blowing into the fire. Next to the fire was a stream of icy water, turbulent and bubbling because the dragons were splashing and jumping in it. A stormy cloud merged with the burning fire and the stream of water. Those who lied under oath or tricked others during their lifetimes were tortured first in the hot fire, then in the ice-cold water, all the time with dragons breathing down their necks. They suffocated in the fire because they had told a lot of lies and they suffered in the cold water, because they had practiced deceit of the darkest kind.

The fire cloud, ice-cold water, and dragons symbolize sicknesses in which patients shiver with fever and chills.

Spiritual Healing

Spiritual healing of lying and cheating needs a lengthy fast, consuming only spelt, vegetables, and fruits, along with the application of a brush massage according to the fasting master. Even people who lie under oath can recover through severe fasting.

The way to truth requires prayer, contemplation, and meditation using such texts as Psalm 51; John 4:23–24, 8:31–32, and 14:6–7; Ephesians 4:14–25 and 5:8–20; and Hebrews 5:11–14.

12. *Contentio*	*Pax*
Contention, war	**Peace**
Strain	Blessedness
Stress	Tranquillity
Tension	Harmony
Conflict	Agreement
Combat	Reconciliation

Crystal Therapy

The gold topaz is used in crystal therapy.

Place a gold topaz on your heart every morning and say the prayer for a strong blessing throughout the day. This ritual gives you inner peace and blesses you with God's own hand so that no evil can befall you (see page 244).

Peace and blessedness are companions, and both are friends of truth. Because truth begins in the womb, pregnant women should avoid the risk factors: contention and unhappiness. Such negative thoughts are absolutely health-destroying for both mother and child. How does Contention look? The fifth apparition has black curly hair and a fiery face. Its many-colored coat has holes and in its hand is an ax. Through its anger the fingers have been cut many times and are splashing blood all over the garment.

Harmful Words of Contention

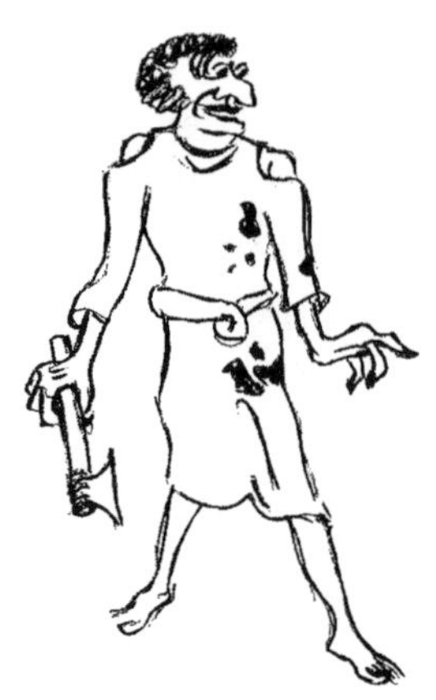

Contention speaks:

"I will not suffer anymore under the great burden of life, like an overloaded donkey. As long as I live and breathe, I will not allow anyone to burden me with his foolish fancies. I will not tolerate being treated like a pile of dirt. I would much rather cause injury to somebody who hurts me. I like to arouse conflict and then fight until my opponent's heart hurts" (LVM).

Healing Words of Peace

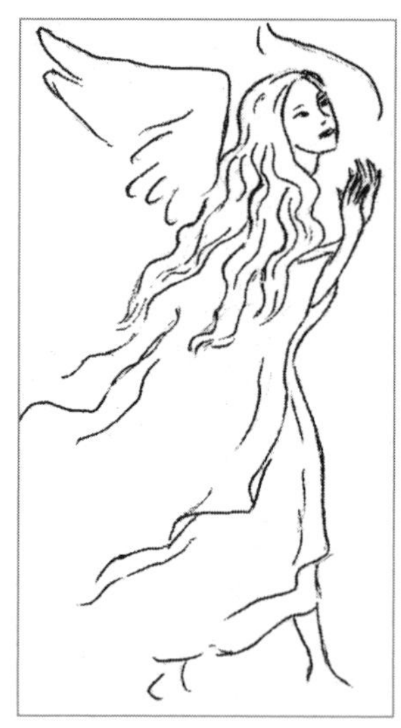

Peacemakers are a remedy for our sick world. They live in inner peace in an atmosphere of incense and myrrh, trying to live their lives without daily stress and struggle. Peace speaks:

"O fire of injuries and insult, you are bloody criminality and the chattering of teeth. Your grievances and hardships cause bloodshed. You boil with rage and want to murder as many friendly and amiable people as possible. Nowhere do you have a home of peace, nor do you have any desire for harmony. You live like a snake in the brush, from where you attack people with your weapons. Like malignant worms [a synonym for viruses] you cause disease and death.

"I am the remedy for all people you damage. I heal what you injure. I disregard your armed forces and war propaganda because I am a mountain of incense and myrrh with the pleasant fragrance of peace. I reside on top of the clouds and attract all that is good. I will thrash you with many strokes as long as you live" (LVM).

Peace is a woman with two wings, one for the good days and one for the bad. She sits on top of the mountains overlooking the conflicts with an atmosphere of innocence:

> I will not endure any tribulations and I want to stay far away from all things contrary to myself. I fear nothing and no one. I will throw down all those who speak evil. I am always joyful and I take my pleasure in all good things. Jesus is the forgiver and consoler of all sorrows, because Jesus endured bodily sorrow [I Peter 2:24]. And because Jesus is just, I wish to join myself to Jesus and to carry him with me. I want to hurl hatred, envy, and all evil things from myself. I also want to have a face that is always joyful in reflecting your justice, O God. (SC III, vision 6:5)

Organ Relationship

Contention, fights, conflicts, and war symbolize the pathology of problems connected with the spinal nerves from the thoracic-lumbar region of the vertebrae, especially Th5. The nervous system of this region controls the gastrointestinal area. Compared to Gluttony, who can eat until bursting, Contention becomes full quickly and suffers from gas and gastro-cardiac pressure. Under extreme pressure from conflict, heart pain can cause a heart attack, especially after a big family dinner or banquet. Contention results typically in disturbances of the entire gastrointestinal function.

Hildegard describes in her medical books virulent worms that cause cancer by their passage from the colon into the blood. The immune system answers the invasion of the viruses with an armada of weapons—free oxygen radicals, for example. The overabundance of free radicals is one of the reasons for the autoaggression of genetic material in the cell nucleus that causes cancer.

Spiritual Healing

Spiritual healing of contention, arguments, and disagreement takes place in the atmosphere of a retreat while fasting. It is important to avoid meat and dairy products. Brush massage and scratchy clothing are also helpful.

The Bible is full of messages about peace, like the famous priestly blessing in Numbers 6:24–26, the praise of the angels in Luke 2:14, Jesus's own words in John 14:27 and 16:32–33, and the words of the apostle Paul in Colossians 3:12–17 and in Philippians 4:4–7.

13. ***Infelicitas*** **Unhappiness**	***Beatitudo*** **Blessedness**
Sadness	Happiness
Depression	Cheerfulness
Blues	Delight
Gloom	Pleasure
Sorrow	Joy
Misery	Rapture

Crystal Therapy

The emerald symbolizes *viriditas* or green power.

Wear the emerald in any form and it will help with all your spiritual and physical weaknesses.

Located on the thirteenth place lie the pair Unhappiness and Blessedness. According to Hildegard, 13 is a lucky number. Unhappiness looks like an outcast with no clothes on. His skin is a mass of contagious scabs. His only covering is leaves and his hands are tearing his chest to pieces.

Harmful Words of Unhappiness

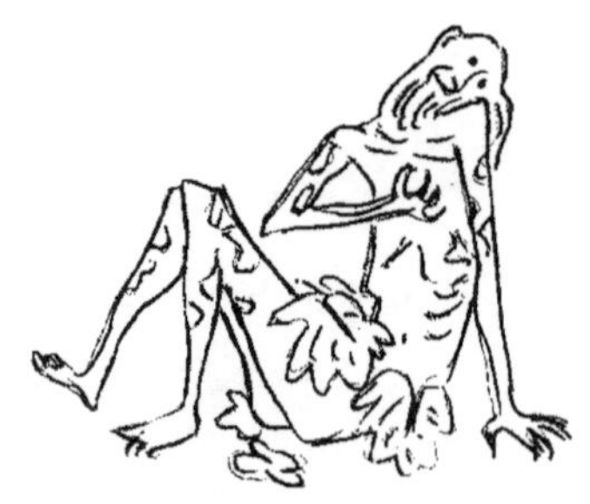

Unhappiness speaks:

"What is my well-being if not my tears? What kind of life do I have other than pain? Who will come to my aid if not death? What answer will come to me other than destruction? There is nothing at all good for me" (LVM).

Healing Word of Blessedness

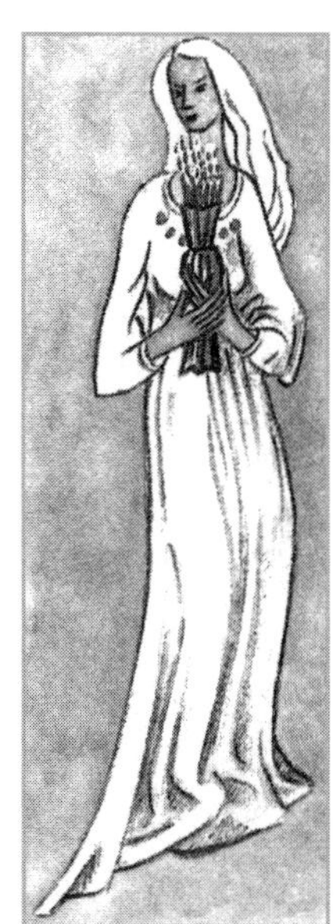

Blessedness answers:

"You chase unhappiness and attract it with pleasure. God has to be called and cherished. You are envious because you have no confidence in God. You don't ask for help and don't receive it. I call him and he answers. I beg for his mercy and he gives what I need. I am full of inner joy. I play the harp in his presence and center all my work around him. I place my faith in God and put my life in his hands. You have no confidence in God and do not yearn for his grace, and that's why you always receive misfortune" (LVM).

Happy is he who can smile about the tragedies in life. Don't give way to despair over disasters in the world; remember, you are blessed.

Blessed are the poor in spirit, for theirs is the kingdom of heaven.
Blessed are those who mourn, for they shall be comforted.
Blessed are the meek, for they shall inherit the earth.
Blessed are those who hunger and thirst for righteousness, for they shall be satisfied.
Blessed are the merciful, for they shall obtain mercy.
Blessed are the pure in heart, for they shall see God.
Blessed are those who are persecuted for righteousness' sake, for theirs is the kingdom of heaven.
Blessed are you when men revile you and persecute you and utter all kinds of evil against you falsely on my account. Rejoice and be glad, for your reward is great in heaven.

—Matthew 5:3–10

Blessedness plays her zither for God:

> I am happy, for Christ Jesus prepares me and makes me beautiful and pure when I flee from the deadly tricks of the devil. The devil is always unhappy in his mind because he has cast God aside and is attracted only to evil works. I flee from this Satan and put him down because he brings me only distress. I desire the lover whom I embrace continuously and whom I hold with joy in all things and above all things. (SC III, vision 6:6)

Organ Relationship

Unhappiness symbolizes the pathology of problems connected with the spinal nerves from the thoracic-lumbar region of the vertebrae, especially Th6. The nervous system of this region controls the gastrointestinal area including digestive organs like the liver, gallbladder, and pancreas. Unhappiness looks like a contagious leper. Skin symptoms always refer to intestinal problems and all skin diseases should be healed from the inside out.

Unhappiness speaks in images of the soul:

> I saw a great ditch with a gigantic width and depth in which there was a burning sulfuric fire full of worms. All people who didn't trust in God during their life were tortured with this fire because they blamed their own nature for all evil. (LVM)

The gastrointestinal infections caused by *Helicobacter pylori* and candida can easily be recognized in the metaphor of burning fire and contagious worms.

Meditation on Truth, Peace, and Happiness

"I am the way and the truth and the life" (John 14:6). This is the theme of all Hildegard's books.

The final goal is always the flow of healing energy from the human soul to the body. This process requires knowledge about the real spiritual risk factors that cause disease. A complete healing in terms of body and soul is possible only if we find the truth about the condition of our soul as summarized in the value system of thirty-five virtues and thirty-five vices. Ask yourself the following questions:

Do I have a problem with vices one to thirty-five? Is my problem money and possessions, anger, bitterness, envy, unhappiness, avarice, depression? Do I expect something good behind every evil? Remember, the soul speaks in symbols and images. Look at the pictures of vices and meditate on the organ relationships and their harmful words. Do I have a problem with the virtues one to thirty-five? Do I need more love, discipline, compassion, patience, truthfulness, peace, or happiness?

As soon as you discover the truth about the condition of your soul, healing energy can flow and the conflict will disappear by itself. Truth, happiness, and peace are inseparable sisters. Happiness is the result of inner peace. Nobody can be happy without truth and peace. The origin of truth, peace, and happiness is the gift of Christmas, when the divine combines with humanity. It is a present for everyone, the poor shepherds and the wealthy kings, and can be observed in the middle of the night. Go out, watch the stars, and listen to their message:

"Glory to God in the highest, and on earth peace to men of good will" (Luke 2:14).

Ask yourself, What is my will? What is my choice? Am I yearning for truth, peace, and happiness? These are the key questions for everybody in all times and everywhere. Christianity has tragically fought for more than two thousand years against evil, and still evil has become more and more powerful like a dragon. If we cut the head of a dragon, he grows ten more heads.

Hildegard called on kings, emperors, and popes, among many others, to understand that the message of Christianity is truth, peace, and happiness, not war, inquisition, and deceit. After all our numerous experiences with wars and fighting, we now know war is the business that makes the most money. All you need is war propaganda and an enemy to get tax money for the war industry. If we understand the lies of war and evil, we can find the truth behind them.

The same is true for the pharmaceutical industry: All you need is a lot of chronically sick patients and drugs with many side effects in order to have permanent consumers. Inner peace and happiness do not require money and possession; they come gratis as a gift, given to you in the symbol of a poor little child in a manger with shepherds grazing their flocks on the fields outside under the stars of a cold winter night.

Spiritual Healing

Spiritual healing of unhappiness takes place when someone really searches for God in solitude or in the peacefulness of the desert. Melancholic people who cannot stay alone should live under the protection and in the refuge of Christian fellowship. Unhappy people are invited to pray the Gold Topaz Prayer (see page 224) from Hildegard every morning, and thereby place their entire lives under the protection of God's blessing.

Bible sources that encourage blessedness and happiness are Psalms 84, 112, and 118:13–29 and the Beatitudes in Matthew 5:3–12.

14. ***Immoderatio*** **Immoderation**	***Discretio*** **Discretion**
Excess	Golden Mean
Overindulgence	Modesty
Exaggeration	Adequacy
Lack of focus	Focus
Uncertainty	Appropriateness
Unreasonable	Reasonable

Crystal Therapy

The jasper helps us concentrate and supports clear thinking.

Place a jasper in your mouth during times of concentration and mental work.

It is no wonder the spirit of immoderation and anarchy follows contention and unhappiness: revolution! Everything, everybody has to be changed, but not I! The seventh character looks like a wolf with crossed legs lying in wait to seize whatever it can. Immoderation celebrates the spirit of anarchy.

Harmful Words of Immoderation

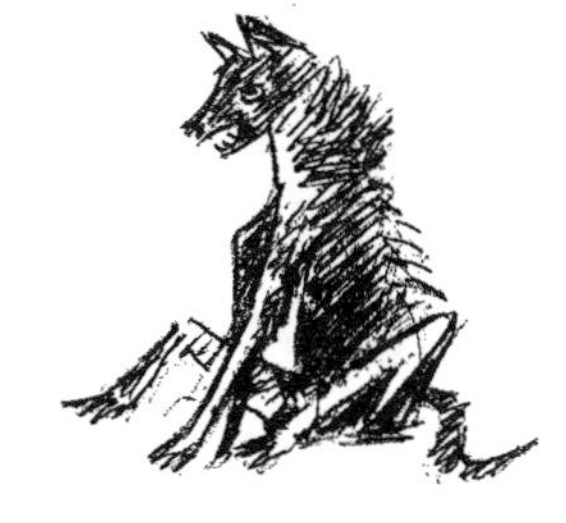

Immoderation speaks:

"Whatever I desire and look for, that I will enjoy. I have no desire to abstain or do without anything. Why should I ignore the needs of my nature? Every physical stimulus is pure pleasure! What is the merit of my life if I live in moderation? I do what I like; fun and games—these are my world. Shall I try to tame my heart when I'm having fun and pleasure? Even if my veins burst from pleasure, I would refuse bloodletting. Why should I be silent when I like to speak? Every stimulus is a spring tonic for me. I live according to my nature. Why change my nature? Everyone should live according to his pleasure" (LVM).

Healing Words of Discretion

Discretion or moderation is a powerful force against the revolutionary spirit. Many people have been transformed in a fundamental way by doing everything in moderation. Moderation answers the immoderate wolf:

"You are sly and deceitful. With your treachery you kill common sense and with your cunning you disturb the harmonic life. You push the extremes like an untrained dog or a mad cow.

"Everything in God's creation has respect for everything else. The stars twinkle from the light of the moon; the moon shines from the sunlight. Everything is related to a greater unity and nothing lives out of its bounds. You do not respect God; you trample and destroy his creation. Your life is wasting away.

"I follow the wanderings of the moon and the orbits of the sun; I explore nature's law. I follow the spirit of charity and compassion. I am a princess in the palace of the king and sparkle like the sunshine. I investigate all his mysteries and I admire his order. You are wounded from your overindulgence and have become food for the malicious worms [viral infection]" (LVM).

Hildegard demonstrates the Golden Mean and its applications by several comparisons:

- Discretion is the balance between the active and the contemplative lifestyle as exemplified in the Benedictine rule *Ora et labora*—that is, somebody who works hard should meditate an equal amount of time. This law is extremely important to a creative life.
- Discretion is like the cornerstone, Jesus, who is the foundation of the entire building of life. This foundation is exemplified by Hildegard's six golden rules—for example, eating and drinking in moderation, sleeping and exercising in appropriate amounts, and caring for the purity of our bodies and our souls.
- Discretion can be compared to a successful businessman who sells good merchandise at a reasonable price.
- Discretion is like the warmth of spring. Spring brings joy and fruits in abundance.
- Discretion is the mother of all values.

Discretion speaks in the book *Scivias:*

> I am the mother of the virtues. I am always looking for the justice of God in all things. I always hope for God to be in my conscience in both spiritual and worldly warfare. I neither condemn nor trample underfoot nor scorn the kings, leaders, protectors, and other worldly magistrates who have been ordained by the author of all things. How can ashes scorn other ashes? The crucified Word of God turned things around for all people, warning them to be just and merciful. Furthermore, I want to hold each and every order and institution in God's world according to his will.
>
> God speaks sometimes to us by touching our hearts and we feel heart pain or cardiac disorder–noticeable in arrhythmia. God speaks through the sweetness of his spirit and gives us the virtues as tools to accomplish his work. No virtue is missing in heaven as well as on earth. God created the firmament, a symbol of the power of discretion, so that man could recognize the spiritual as well as the fleshly necessities. We shall look for both: the yearning for eternity and the caring for physical needs. Live by the Golden Mean. Don't build a ruin through exaggeration, or ruin yourself with excessive desire. We shall sigh and pray, fulfilling good deeds at

> an appropriate time and caring for our daily needs at another. Try hard and exercise daily—regardless of what charismatic gifts you have. Moderation prevents vanity; it is a horror for God, as extravagance serves only you and not God. (SC III, vision 6:7)

Hildegard writes: "I saw a great ocean from unlimited depth and breadth burning with an immense sulfuric fire. All people who lived in immoderation and excess during their lifetimes were tortured in this fire" (LVM).

Bloodletting

Hildegard's medicine has an extremely important remedy to cleanse the blood. The purging of blood and the lymphatic humors is the prerequisite for good health, as blood nourishes the entire body. Bloodletting is a well-established method in traditional medicine to cleanse the blood and stimulate the immune system. Simultaneously the entire metabolism comes into balance—for example, cholesterol, blood pressure, and the viscosity of the blood—to prevent stroke or heart attack.

Every physician is trained to take blood. If he or she follows Hildegard's rules, miracles will occur!

- Take blood only after the full moon and six days thereafter.
- The patient should not eat or drink before bloodletting.
- Let the blood flow and stop when its color changes from black to red, approximately 150 to a maximum of 200 ml.
- Follow a Hildegard diet after bloodletting, and avoid sunshine and computer and TV screens for three days.
- Bloodletting should occur once a year; in severe cases of sickness, twice a year may be necessary.

Organ Relationship

Immoderation and excess symbolize the pathology of problems connected with the spinal nerves from the thoracic-lumbar region of the vertebrae, especially Th7. The nervous system of this region controls the gastrointestinal area including such digestive organs as the liver, gallbladder, and pancreas. Excess in eating and drinking as well as a stressful lifestyle cause bad humors and disease.

Meditation on Discretion

According to the second day of creation, "And God made the firmament and separated the waters which were under the firmament from the waters which were above the firmament. And it was so" (Genesis 1:7).

The firmament symbolizes the golden separation line of discretion, which separates the active daily life, *vita activa,* from the celestial life of contemplation, *vita contemplativa.* Discretion is like a golden stairway climbing into heaven through good works and descending to earth in order to stand with both feet on the ground. Both parts of life are full of joy, because God is the founder. Hildegard writes:

> The power of discretion helps to bring everything to a good end. God has also foreseen that the beginning has a happy end, as a good work is useless without accomplishment. All virtues have a heavenly and an earthly part, because we live on earth and still look up into the sky.

Hildegard calls the power of discretion "heaven in humanity." Just as all the beauty on earth is illuminated from the firmament, so do all the virtues radiate in humanity. Body and soul are both under the direct control of discretion. Discretion is an important value portrayed in the second day of creation.

> The firmament supports all the stars and planets with the help of discretion like an operator and in the same manner discretion is also the main operator for all the virtues. (LDO, vision 5:29)

Spiritual Healing

Spiritual healing of immoderation, overindulgence, and extravagance requires abstinence from animal proteins as in fatty cheese, meat, and dairy products in exchange for a modest diet with spelt, fruits, and vegetables.

The afflicted who seek moderation and discretion will find help reading and meditating on the following Bible passages: Psalm 25, Proverbs 2:1–11, Ephesians 4:1–6, and I Peter 5:5–11.

15. ***Perditio animarum***	***Salvatio animarum***
Lost soul	**Saved soul**
Doom	Salvation
Destruction	Healing
Damnation	Redemption, rescue
Misery	Well-being
Distance to God	Identity with God
Ruin	Tower of God

Crystal Therapy

The emerald contains the healing power for salvation and can be used for all spiritual and physical weaknesses.

The color green stands for green energy, or *viriditas,* which Hildegard sees as the flowing power behind all creation. Wear the emerald in a ring or on a necklace.

The previous vices destroy the basis of human nature and plunge the soul into a state of despair and decay. At some time every one of us is caught in a condition of lost energy and exhaustion, which can lead to infirmities and the final state of death.

Harmful Words of Doom

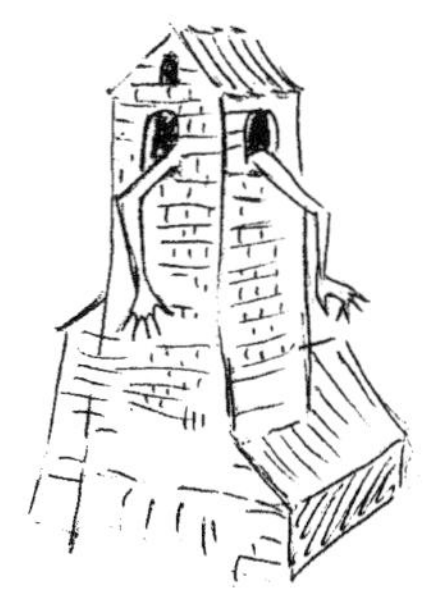

The lost soul looks like a ruin with three windows. A flat roof blocks the view to the sky. A cadaver stretches two arms out the window and speaks:

"What merits and reward do I have? Only the burning fire! My whole being and I cry forever. I flee from the radiant beauty of life and refuse to accomplish good works. I hate radiance and the splendor of light, because I, the body snatcher, am there to plunder souls. That's my profession and my duty, for I come from Satan. I am his disgrace and damnation" (LVM).

Healing Words of Salvation

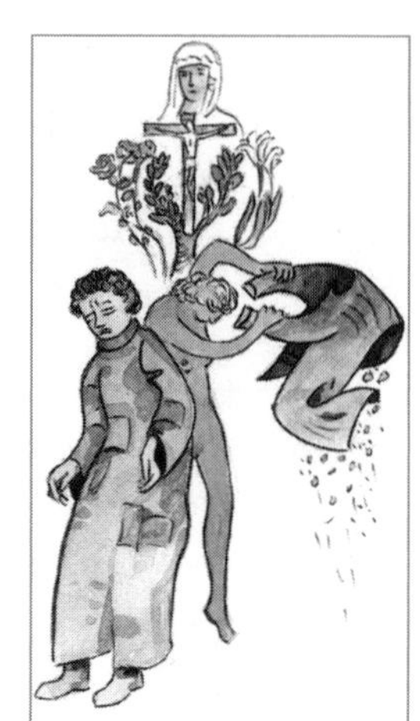

Salvation answers:

"You are Satan's arrow who flies through the night. You kill the favored few who think differently from you. You strive for destruction, but the blessed fight with the angels against you and try to drown you. Just as during the great flood, they will flood you with baptism and the power of the gifts of the Holy Spirit: wisdom, piety, and strength. That will be your end, because you are an enemy against God.

"I am a castle filled with all values and a protective tower for Jerusalem built from the works of the saints. I recognize those in misery and despair, like the ram in the burning bush. I save and heal the depraved by salvation through baptism and the power of God. I am cured through the radiant power of Jesus and walk together with God" (LVM).

The closer we are to God, the more energy flows. Because nobody is free from anxiety, each of us looks for protection and security. That's why insurance companies are so powerful. Nevertheless, only trust in God enables us to survive and gain his infinite power to change and regenerate. That is the lesson for the lost soul. If anarchy is not restored to former happiness and peace, life turns into slavery.

Organ Relationship

Doom, perdition, damnation, despair, depravity, and decay symbolize the pathology of problems connected with the spinal nerves from the thoracic-lumbar region of the vertebrae, especially Th8. The nervous system of this region controls the intestinal area, including the pathology of excretion from the kidneys and the colon. Urine and feces are the end products of digestion and should be eliminated. We suffer terribly from self-poisoning if something goes wrong. "Death comes from the colon"—Hildegard describes 850 years before our time how the body commits suicide in the form of autoaggression. The three windows of the ruin symbolize the three parts of the digestive tract—the stomach, intestines, and colon—with their corresponding sicknesses.

Perdition, damnation, and despair can provoke satanic pain. People who live in despair create infernal pain, because they do not trust in God.

Meditation on Salvation

Salvation is the power of God. The power of salvation carries us in critical situations and brings us from the paradise of our mother's womb into the reality of our daily lives, from birth to death. Childbirth is a miracle! In 99 percent of all cases, no doctor is needed. Childbirth has been happening under nature's protection without medication, without an episiotomy, and without anesthesia for the past forty thousand years. If we collaborate with nature, we have the greatest security. If we leave or forget nature, we have the highest risk.

Sage Tea

Salvation is in Latin salvere, *or "to heal." Hildegard says, "I save and I heal."* Salvia officinalis *is sage. Sage tea cleanses noxious and toxic material from our blood.*

Place 1 teaspoon of sage leaves in 1 cup of water and boil for 1 minute. Remove the plant material. Drink 1 cup a day for 4 weeks. This is very effective against cystitis.

Every one of us is a child of God and belongs inseparably to the salvation program of nature. The baby is equipped with everything it needs to survive. It is entrusted with the treasure of fifteen healing powers to stay healthy. The number 15 is the total of 3 times 5 and symbolizes a unity of body, soul, and mind. All the other spiritual forces will be acquired later in life—during childhood and adolescence, numbers 16–22; in adulthood, numbers 23–30; and even in old age we learn five new lessons, numbers 31–35.

The spiritual forces from conception (numbers 1–7) and from pregnancy (numbers 8–15) substantially influence the prenatal value system. This program keeps us healthy, happy, whole, and holy because all of us are under the protection of the divine. It is good to remember that each of us—even those with a predisposition for weakness and sickness acquired during conception or pregnancy—is equipped with the same wonderful golden soul containing the divine and cosmic forces. If we live in harmony with nature and ourselves, our soul can do something to keep us healthy, whole, and holy.

Spiritual Healing

Spiritual healing for the lost soul far from God occurs by learning how to trust in God, through fasting, nightly meditation, and giving aid to the poor. Nobody knows the soul unless he believes in God. Trust occurs when we open our eyes for the miracles that are hidden in nature: "Everything that is created by God contains a miracle, which nobody knows unless it is revealed to him or her from God."

Bible passages like the following can be a help during prayer and meditation: Psalms 34, 109:21–31, and 130; Daniel 3:17–18; Luke 19:10; Colossians 1:9–14; and I Timothy 1:12–20.

Chapter 5

The Northman

Infancy: The Third Section from Hip to Knee

At the moment we are born we are entrusted with all the information we need to travel through life. We are already equipped with the harmonious partnership of a visible body that contains more than 100,000 cellular genes and an invisible soul with its thirty-five spiritual powers to master life. But to our great astonishment, we are completely helpless and require our parents to take care of and support us.

At this stage of childhood we must go through the seven lessons of humility, charity, respect for God, obedience, faith, hope, and chastity as guidelines for the journey through life accompanied by spiritual growth. In order to gain these values, we need to face the reality that values have to be developed and acquired by our own efforts.

Spiritual training must overcome many hard experiences like failures, mistakes, disappointments, frustrations, hurts, sicknesses, and setbacks. The best way to learn the seven childhood virtues is by overcoming their opposites—arrogance, envy, thirst for fame, disobedience, infidelity, desperation, and luxury. The weaknesses in our lives are opportunities to see the transforming power behind them, so that sickness leads to health, an enemy becomes a friend, and nonsense has a deeper meaning leading us to sense and wisdom. The purpose in life is not to fight against evil in human nature but instead to understand its message and use the evil as a chance for personal spiritual growth.

The Acquired Virtues of Childhood

In the second group of virtues and vices, dominated by pregnancy and motherhood, the mother is responsible for inherited virtues and vices. Now, the third group deals with the virtues and vices acquired through education during childhood. The outcome of a fulfilled life depends heavily on the engagement of both parents. Children without the experience of humility, supportive relationships, and love during infancy find it difficult to pass on the same virtues later in life. Children need dedicated fathers and mothers in order to develop into adulthood. Indigenous people all over the world used to have a specific education for young boys and girls to become strong men and women. The Aborigines of central Australia, for example, used very tough initiation ceremonies with occasional pain over a period of a decade to educate their children.

Our Western society, with its lack of initiation ceremonies, is ill prepared to educate its own children, and that's why the generations clash.

The seven virtues in this group are necessary to educate children so that they may grow up free and with respect for their fellow man.

The third region is under control of the autonomic nervous system. The delicate interplay of sex hormones and the autonomic nervous system stimulates the reproduction system and all organs and muscles in this area, including sexuality. During infancy we must acquire the seven virtues that influence the proper functioning of this area.

16. *Superbia* (arrogance)	*Humilitas* (humility)
17. *Invidia* (envy)	*Charitas* (charity)
18. *Inanis gloria* (thirst for glory)	*Timor Domini* (reverence for God)

19. *Inobedientia* (disobedience)	*Obedientia* (obedience)
20. *Infidelitas* (lack of faith)	*Fides* (faith)
21. *Desperatio* (despair)	*Spes* (hope)
22. *Luxuria* (obscenity)	*Castitas* (chastity)

16. *Superbia*	***Humilitas***
Arrogance	**Humility**
Egoism	Modesty
Conceit	Simplicity
Vanity	Naturalness

Crystal Therapy

The amethyst strengthens a weak personality in times of humiliation.

Whoever is influenced negatively by his environment (colleagues or claustrophobia, for example) should wear an amethyst boldly and conspicuously.

Humility is the power that lifts us after great disappointments. A legend from Saint Francis of Assisi exemplifies admirable humility. While he was walking with a friend over snowfields in order to celebrate Christmas in his cloister, Saint Francis asked, "What is the greatest joy in life?" The friend replied, "See the cloister in the distance? Pretty soon we will knock on the door and our brothers will welcome us to celebrate with them. That's the greatest joy in the world!"

"No," responded Saint Francis, "totally wrong. The greatest joy in life is when we knock on the door and our friends kick us out in the dark shouting: 'Go to hell, you beggars.' If you can laugh in spite of that, you have the power of humility."

Arrogance, its opposite, is way up high before the downfall that leads to humility. Arrogance is the beginning of all malignancy and its first manifestation is in Lucifer, who wanted to be better and greater than God.

Arrogance is one of the classical vices, and it cannot be cured by fasting;

on the contrary, fasting may increase an arrogant attitude. Arrogance has burning eyes and a nose full of filth, but no arms or hands. Instead it has wings like a bat and speaks out of the darkness, a symbol for the media (such as radio and newspapers) transmitting propaganda.

Harmful Words of Arrogance

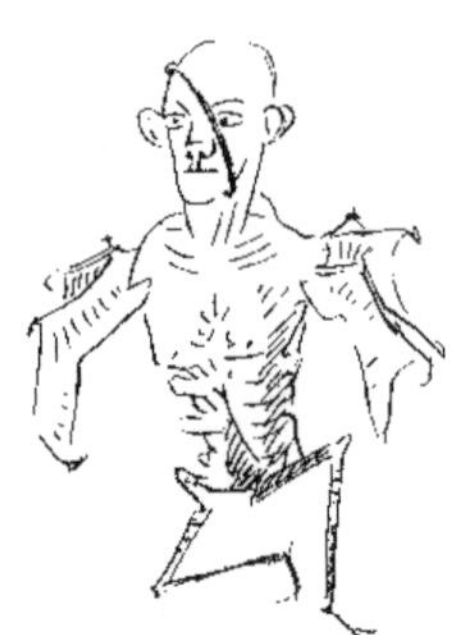

The voice of Arrogance:

"My voice screams far over the mountains. Who is greater than I am? I spread my mantle over all the hills and fields and want nobody to offer resistance. No one is greater than I" (LVM).

Healing Words of Humility

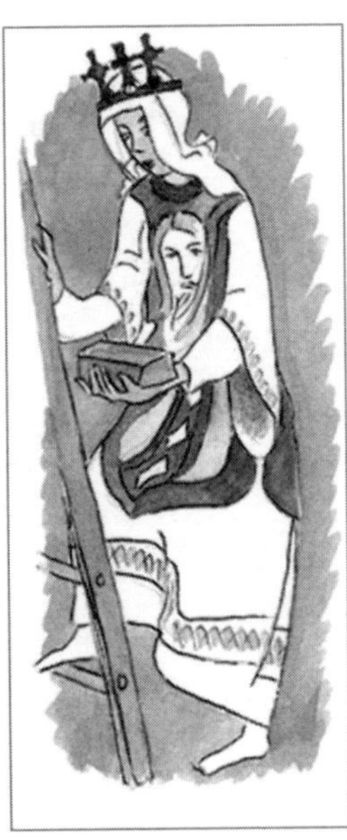

Humility responds:

"I am just like the white cumulus cloud. Why should I suffer if someone injures me with great injustice? Even the Creator descended from heaven to embrace his beloved human. I, Humility, was with the Creator in heaven descending with him. I live all over the earth. I cannot glorify myself to become something special; otherwise, I would not be the sun that shines in the dark. With the help of God, I penetrate all blackness on earth and in the universe" (LVM).

Also, "Why shouldn't I be happy when somebody beats me with injustice? The Son of God himself descended from heaven to embrace humanity. I, Humility, was with him in

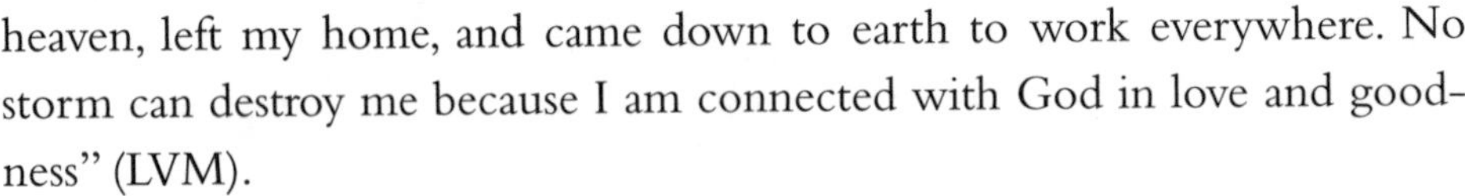

heaven, left my home, and came down to earth to work everywhere. No storm can destroy me because I am connected with God in love and goodness" (LVM).

Humility is the queen of the virtues in Hildegard's miracle play *Ordo virtutem* and leads the soul back to God.

> I am Humility, the pillar of humble minds and the assassin of proud hearts. I began in the least of places, but I have ascended to the lofty

> heavens. Lucifer lifted himself upward, but fell downward. Whoever wishes to imitate me and desires to be my child, and if that person wants to embrace me as if I were his mother by doing my work, let this person touch the ground and then gently lift himself to the top.

"What does this mean? Let this person think about the weakness of his own flesh, and let this person climb step by step upward from virtue to virtue with a sweet and gentle spirit. Whoever climbs first to the highest branch of a tree most often falls unexpectedly. But whoever begins by climbing from the base of the tree will not fall so easily if he proceeds cautiously" (SC III, vision 8:1).

Organ Relationship

Arrogance, self-love, egoism, vanity, haughtiness, selfishness, and conceit relate to the pathology of problems connected with the spinal nerves from the thoracic-lumbar region of vertebrae Th9 (humility) to L3 (chastity). The nervous system here controls the liver, gallbladder, pancreas, kidneys, suprarenal glands, descending colon, and rectum as well as the urogenital organs. Inflammation of these organs can cause severe autoaggressive diseases including hepatitis, cholecystitis, pancreatitis, nephritis, colitis, hemorrhoids, cancer, AIDS, multiple sclerosis, and polyarthritis. Such inflammations usually end with the suffix *-itis.*

Meditation on Humility

Humility is quite stable, but its opposite—arrogance—often causes headfirst falls and crashes. Arrogance is the demon of pride. Humility is for Hildegard the force that gives us the strength to cope with our daily lives, in poor or bad times, through offenses and disease. More, though, humility is the power to enjoy life even in times of hardship, like disappointment, personal loss, sickness, injury, distress, harm, pain, grief, or cruel treatment. We learn to be realistic with Hildegard. She always emphasizes that our normal life is a battleground, full of conflicts and tragedy, and yet we always have the freedom to decide on which side we struggle.

Humility is the power to overcome failure and sickness, a chance to become empowered with spirituality and joy. We remain in arrogance and self-love, stay haughty and selfish in our daily lives, unless the echo of our souls forces us to stop and return to modesty and humility. Hildegard writes that our humiliations of little consequence in comparison with those of Jesus Christ, the Son of God, who died like a criminal.

Hildegard describes the result of arrogance and conceit in symbols related to fire and embers caused by stinging worms (LVM).

Spiritual Healing

Spiritual healing for arrogance, egoism, and conceit comes from humility. Begin by bending your knees while sighing and crying. Put on scratchy clothes and use a brush massage. Fasting is not recommended in this case, as fasting creates a feeling of success and superiority, which is not helpful for arrogant people.

Meditate on the spirit of humility with the following Bible passages: Isaiah 66:2b, Matthew 11:29, Ephesians 4:2–6, and James 4:6–10.

17. *Invidia* — *Charitas*

Envy	**Charity**
Jealousy	Self-esteem
Selfishness	Oneness with others
Self-centeredness	Oneness with God
Rivalry	Cooperation
Malevolence, bitterness	Benevolence
Holding a grudge	Fairness
Aversion	Sympathy
Resentment	Kindness

Crystal Therapy

The amethyst helps establish good relationships, especially in a hostile atmosphere.

If you are influenced negatively by your environment (colleagues or claustrophobia, for example), wear an amethyst boldly and conspicuously.

Charity is the power that keeps us in harmonious relationship with ourselves, with others, and with God.

Social relationships are essential to maintain health and happiness. Charity is the power that keeps energy flowing among God, others, and ourselves. With charity we tap into the energy of God, because God is the source of charity that weaves all life in a divine ecological architectural tapestry. Charity enables all the relations to flow smoothly.

Charity and love accompany days of joy, but even more the dark days of sickness, misery, and calamity. Charity enables us to tolerate and forgive the imperfections of others and of ourselves. Love and charity open our eyes to the good behind the evil, to find a cure for sickness, to experience support for problems.

Hildegard's concept of charity has many forms and manifestations. One of them she calls *amor caritatis,* which includes erotic love and respect for one other. This love creates optimal conditions during the conception of a new baby. She explains that children who are conceived with *amor caritatis* will be healthy, talented, and gifted with virtues. This concept of love is quite the opposite of Hollywood's love, where it is degraded to pure sex, a product to buy. Sex without love has become an addiction in our modern society and kills a harmonious relationship. The absence of charity makes people envious and promotes selfish, egoistic, and materialistic reactions.

The connection between charity and envy is not always obvious unless we understand that charity incorporates the needs of others, whereas envy ignores and resents others. More, though, envy sees only its own advantage, is selfish, and pampers its ego. Envy has an ugly brother—hate.

Envy is a hideous monster with bear claws, wooden feet, and a fiery red head.

Harmful Words of Envy

With a flame of fire, Envy speaks:

"I am the shepherd and protector of every excess. I extinguish the life energy in every human being. I suppress all common sense, wisdom, and intelligence. I damage everybody and everything. I manipulate and command all people and destroy God's creation.

"If I cannot own beauty and goodness," at least I will drag it into the mud. Even if some hate me like the darkness, I shall always return. I send out my flattering words like arrows in the dark and hurt all good-hearted people. The north wind is my destructive power. Everything I do, I do out of hate for humanity, because hatred grows out of me even though hatred is inferior to me" (LVM).

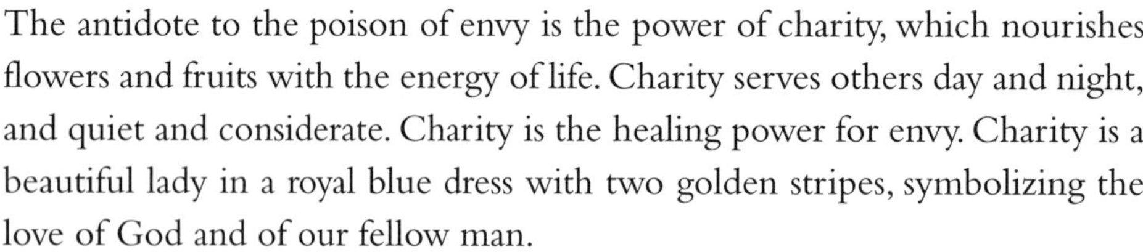

The antidote to the poison of envy is the power of charity, which nourishes flowers and fruits with the energy of life. Charity serves others day and night, and quiet and considerate. Charity is the healing power for envy. Charity is a beautiful lady in a royal blue dress with two golden stripes, symbolizing the love of God and of our fellow man.

Healing Words of Charity

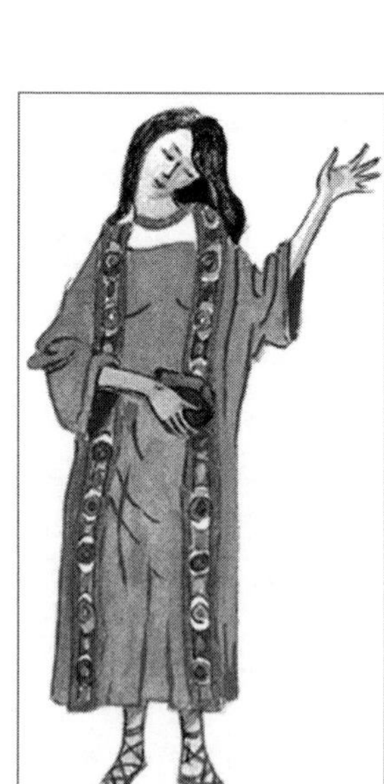

Charity fights against Envy:

"O filthy trickster, you are like a snake committing suicide. You lack stability and respect. You are like an idol fighting against God, killing people with falsehood and deceit. You call yourself hell, the infernal region without love. You destroy everything coming out of God's wisdom, even beautiful, radiant life.

"I am the air that nourishes everything with green life energy and brings forth flowers and fruits. My teacher is the Holy Spirit, who generates the strongest flow of love from God to me. This enables me to do good deeds through my tears. I am the mild rain that lets herbs and flowers grow in joy.

"You, Envy, are a strong poison that works against a person's essential nature, but you cannot destroy it. The more you rage, the more you provoke the beauty and power of God's flower garden and vineyard. . . . I create by day and by night the power of equality, serenity, and symmetry. With my shield I protect everybody. I invigorate good deeds during the day and regenerate the body at night. I am the sweetest friend of God and take part in his decisions. Everything that belongs to God belongs to me, because I am a part of God. I heal wounds as the Son of God heals sins. You should be ashamed of yourself, because you are the opposite of love" (LVM).

We have to accept that love in its three dimensions is the keystone of life. In the search for happiness, love is the energy that holds the universe in harmony. The three forces of love are balanced in the classic triangle of God, the others (family, friends, neighbors, and so on), and oneself.

In the Middle Ages, love of God became the official worldview and religion a powerful instrument of the church, declaring every opposing opinion to be heresy or treason. Hildegard emphasizes that love is a power existing in an eternal realm. The only way we can reach that realm is to tap into God's energy by prayer and thus bring it down to earth.

Hildegard writes:

> I, Charity, am in the incarnate Word of God descended to earth, where a multitude of faithful people—armed with just and good skills—have been made perfect through me. . . . O Humility, you have lifted right up to the stars those trampled on and saddened. O Humility, you who are the most glorious queen of the virtues, you are a strong and unconquerable defense force. Those who choose you with a pure heart do not fall down. (SC III, vision 8:2)

Humanity becomes instructed through the teacher, the Holy Spirit, with the wisdom of God, centered in the law of charity.

Writes Hildegard: "We shall place all our trust in God and treat others as we would like to be treated. Charity can reach the core of people and change our lives as well as the entire universe. Our well-being depends on charity.

Stars are shining in the sky for the orientation of the people. They send us the power of the virtue charity to illuminate the dark side of our existence so we will not break under the burden of our daily life. The stars are strong signs looking up to God and teaching us to ask for help and support."

Organ Relationship

Envy, jealousy, rivalry, hated, ill will, aversion, antipathy, indignation, and bitterness are connected to the pathology of the nervous system from the thoracic-lumbar region of the vertebrae Th10 to L3. This region influences the liver, gallbladder, pancreas, kidneys, suprarenal glands, colon, and rectum as well as the urogenital organs. Here lie the causes of autoaggression and inflammation of the stomach and intestinal system as well as of the inner organs.

Hildegard sees in her vision of Envy a mountain full of scorpions producing inner freezing, just like a fit of shivering during an infection (LVM).

Meditation on Cosmos and Charity

Hildegard's powerful text on cosmos and charity opens a window not only to the function of the universe but also to the miracle of the Holy Spirit becoming material as it operates in the universe. We are able to understand that the Spirit is the source and origin of all life, including the life of the universe, which Hildegard regards as a living organism. *Caritas*—Charity, the marvelous bride of the Spirit—is the innermost life-giving part of creation. She "nourishes all green, brings forth life, is filled with the breath of the Spirit," and sings:

Caritas habundat in omnia

Charity is abundant in all things,
from the depths to the heights,
above the highest stars,
and is most loving to all things;
for to the high king
it has given the kiss of peace.

Charity is the love who sings the Songs of Songs, which Hildegard calls a "Symphonia harmoniae celestium revelationum" to indicate that the cosmos is established in harmony. Sun, moon, and stars hold their places in harmonious revolution since the beginning of time. Everything is set up in celestial beauty and perfection, in love and cosmic harmony.

Music, the harmonious manifestation of human activity, connects us to the music of cosmic charity, which sings with the stars, planets, and other moving spheres. "During rotation the firmament emits a marvelous sound that we cannot hear, because of its height and its largeness," Hildegard writes in *Causae et Curae.*

The Universe Is Harmony

We can make audible the sound of the earth by calculating its audio frequency. To receive the frequency per second, we divide 1 by the revolution time of the planet in seconds. Everything on earth lives in harmony with the vibration of Mother Earth. She rotates around herself in exactly 23 hours, 56 minutes, and 2 seconds.

Flowers open to the sunlight and close at night. Trees, birds, and even precious stones vibrate in resonance with the earth and we all wake up, sleep, work, and live according to the rotation of the earth. Even our genetic code, our DNA, vibrates in resonance with the 24-hour frequency of the earth, which also keeps it alive.

THE SOUND OF THE EARTH

We can increase our resonance with Mother Earth when we make the sound of the earth audible and visible. All we have to do is divide 1 by the number of seconds in 23 hours, 56 minutes, and 2 seconds, which is $^1/_{86,164}$ seconds, which equals a frequency of 0.000 0016 cycles per second. This frequency is of course inaudible, but if we multiply with 24 octaves we can hear the higher frequency of 194.7 Hertz, which is the sound of G, the key sound of the violin system. The name in French is *sol,* which means "soil, ground" or even *soleil,* for the sun in resonance with the earth. We can make the earth sound visible by multiplying with 65 octaves to see the color bright orange with a frequency of 428 million Hertz or 700 nanometers. We can meditate to the earth sound G in a bright orange light in order to increase the resonance with mother earth and be in tune with the entire universe as well as with the atoms in the microcosm, speaking: "I love the earth; I receive the power of the earth."

THE SOUND OF THE SUN

The earth travels 365.242 days around the sun, which equals 31,556,926 seconds. If we multiply this frequency by 32 octaves, we can hear a tone with 136.10 Hertz, which is a *cis* in the chromatic scale. The *cis* sound is in India, Tibet, and Japan the sound of light, the father of sounds. This tone causes geraniums to blossom in winter. Temple bells and gongs vibrate with this sound. The sound of the sun fills us with light when we meditate: "I am light" or "Let us walk in the light of the Lord."

Amazing pictures from the space telescope Hubbell reveal today what Hildegard saw 850 years ago. These photographs correspond harmoniously to Hildegard's beautiful cosmic illuminations and show the fire-red nature of the gift of charity and the interstellar galaxies.

There is abundant love in the world soul of the universe transferred to us as music when we dance and sing. Love is an energy that keeps us alive. Love others and return to God, because he is the source and origin of all love.

AN EXERCISE IN CHARITY

This exercise promotes the power of love and charity.

Take Hildegard's illumination of the cosmic man and stand, as he does, on the tips of your toes. Stretch your hands toward the sun. Inhale and enjoy the stretching of the muscles in your legs. Go back down on your feet and stay on the ground while you exhale. Relax and hold your hands in front of you to form a bowl. Look into this bowl and speak, "I am ready to receive." Open your hands and stretch again and speak, "I am ready to give."

Spiritual Healing

Spiritual healing of envy and jealousy requires the therapeutic effort and push of charity and love. We become loving when we toughen our bodies with fitness, wear scratchy clothing, and begin the day with a ritual combination of brush massage before we shower and exercise and meditation preceding going off to work.

Fasting is not recommended in this case.

Practice meditation and prayer using the words from Deuteronomy 6:4–9; Psalms 33, 86, 103, and 118; and the famous passage about love in I Corinthians 13.

18. *Inanis gloria*	*Timor Domini*
Thirst for glory	**Reverence for God**
Thirst for fame	Veneration
Celebrity, hero worship	Reverence
Worship of idols	Worship and fear of God
Bragging	Adoration

Crystal Therapy

The green emerald contains *viriditas,* or life energy, and reminds us of the presence of God's energy during every instant of our lives.

Wear the emerald set in a ring or on a chain.

Fear of God is the power that lifts us up when we are prisoners of our own habits and desires. If we disrespect the divine center in our souls, we lose our roots and begin to look for other idols, such as drugs, alcohol, and work.

Thirst for glory is a companion of envy. As soon as someone is envious of of his neighbor's status or prestige, he wants to be famous himself. Hildegard describes this vanity as a conductor dressed in his dark tailcoat and waving flowers over his head. His hat, made out of grass, is a symbol of his thirst for fame and appreciation. The black color signifies the brief, fleeting character of his fame.

Harmful Words of Thirst for Glory

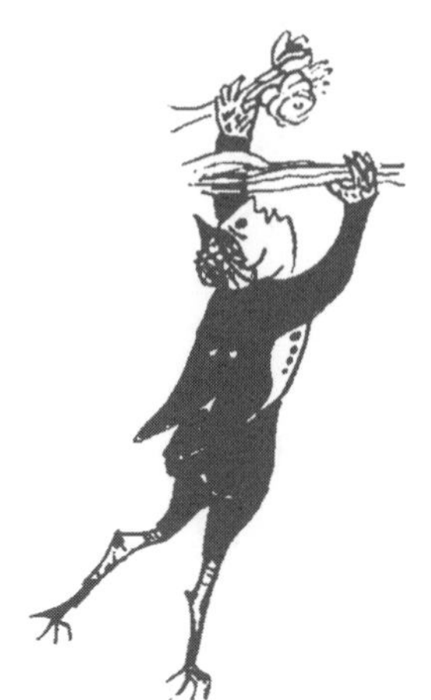

Thirst for Glory speaks:

"I'm always looking out for my own benefit and my own interests. I have so much confidence in myself that I can fly with my own publicity campaign through villages and countrysides just as do the birds. The propaganda of my campaign can change the image of a wild monster into the charm of a young girl.

"I organize everything that is mine so well that all who see me will be pleased and all who hear me will grant me honor and glory. Everybody will wonder about such an example of giving one's best" (LVM).

Healing Words of Reverence for God

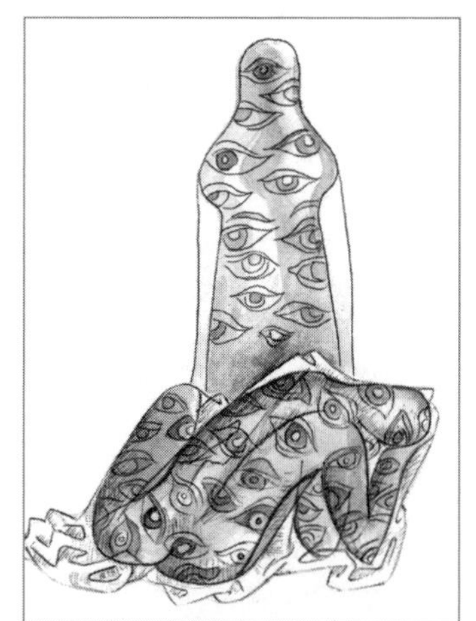

Reverence for God responds:

"You have no respect for anything and always put yourself in the center of interest. You are empty, because God is missing in your thinking; you are your own God. But nobody achieves anything without God's grace. All your gifts and talents come from God."

God kills everybody who turns the wheel of God's knowledge around his own glorification. But if you ask for help, God is on your side. If you work without him and are concerned only with your own interests, God will turn you down. When you reject salvation and the remedies of God (which are the spiritual and medicinal remedies of Hildegard's healing art), you are far from real life.

"But I, Reverence for God, stand up straight and am responsible for my thoughts and deeds. I make nothing special out of my deeds, and I fulfill what God expects. I sigh in love to God and respect God's order and judgment. I will have my reward in eternity. This is possible only if I stay away from the smell of sin, the glamour of the world, and the addiction of the flesh by trying to stay free.

"I respect God's creation and go in peace with all people. God gives me the breath of life, and no matter how many obstacles block my way, I will continuously fulfill my duty. God provided the foundations in the human race to build a home under his protection. Remember this and speak about it to others.

"Your thirst for fame is a farce; your destiny and fate, no honor at all" (LVM)!

Everybody is somehow responsible for others in life (lovers, parents, managers, for example) and needs guidance from a higher power. Moses was responsible for his people and had to lead them for forty years through the desert to their homeland. He had no lighthouse and no compass but God, who showed him the way as a cloud during the day and a fire column during the night. Respect for God is the best guide through life and helps you not to get lost.

Writes Hildegard:

> I am Reverence for God. O woe to the wretched sinners who do not respect God but instead consider God a deceiver! Who is able to flee the fear of God? God allows the guilty, who do not hurl evil things away from themselves, to perish. I stand in great awe of God! Who will free me from God's fearsome judgment? No one except the one just God. Therefore, I will seek that one God, I will always flee to that one God. (SC III, vision 8:3)

Organ Relationship

Thirst for glory and celebrity, idol worship, and bragging relate to the pathology of the nervous system in the region of Th11. This area governs the visceral organs—the liver, pancreas, and kidneys—and the intestinal system. This section is also responsible for energizing the female and male sex organs. (See Frank H. Netter, *Atlas of Human Anatomy*.)

In her vision Hildegard sees a vast swamp full of worms, gas, and bad smells causing inflammation and autoaggression like gastritis and colitis in addition to hepatitis, nephritis, pancreatitis, and/or urogenital disorders (LVM).

MOMENTS OF WONDER AND AWE

The invisible God becomes visible in his creation especially where there is higher natural strength and power, called vortex energy. This energy has a great healing influence on every creature, from human beings and animals to plants. Vortex energy is found in secret and sacred ceremonial places and in areas with a positive influence on the wellness of their populations.

Places with strong energy exist at the ocean's shore and atop mountains and hills. This energy makes it possible to be mentally uplifted to higher levels of consciousness. In combination with a meditation on sunrise or on sunset, the vortex energy becomes a spiritual boost for power, advancement, and enlightenment. The Rocky Mountains, the Grand Canyon, and the Red Hills of Sedona, Arizona, make ideal places for a spiritual retreat, especially when you enter these areas full of respect for God and his Creation.

Other situations of awe and worship can be enjoyed throughout the year—during the change of the seasons, in a thunderstorm, at the sight of a rainbow. The birth of a child, a wedding, even a funeral can be moments of unforgettable emotion and reverence. Many people find the presence of God when they are alone in the stillness.

Spiritual Healing

Spiritual healing of thirst for glory or for fame requires the therapeutic effort of trembling fear of, respect for, and worship of God combined with reverence, esteem, and admiration for nature. We become respectful and reverent when we proceed to fast, strengthen our bodies with fitness and sauna in combination with brush massage before each shower, and work out with hard physical exercise.

We can control our thirst for glory with daily prayer and meditation, as with the words of Psalms 92, 96, 98, and 100.

19. ***Inobedientia***	***Obedientia***
Disobedience	**Obedience**
Insolence, disrespect	Respect
Defiance	Compliance
Resistance	Cooperation
Impertinence	Adaptability
Rebellion	Friendship

Crystal Therapy

The sardonyx helps sharpen the intellect, increases wisdom, and encourages obedience and understanding of others.

Wear the sardonyx as a necklace or bracelet and lick the stone occasionally. This will sharpen all five senses.

Obedience is the power of listening to each other and consequently taking part in the harmony of the universe. The result is comparable to the harmony of a symphony orchestra in which more than eighty musicians play different instruments but still speak one language. In addition, obedience is the art of understanding the language of God and fulfilling his will.

Disobedience is a form of egoism whereby the person pursues his own happiness at the cost of others. Disobedience is a risk factor for life on this planet and causes much harm and damage both to the created order and to nature.

Disobedience has the head of a snake, the legs and feet of a viper, and the body of a crab, and shakes and rocks from head to toe.

Harmful Words of Disobedience

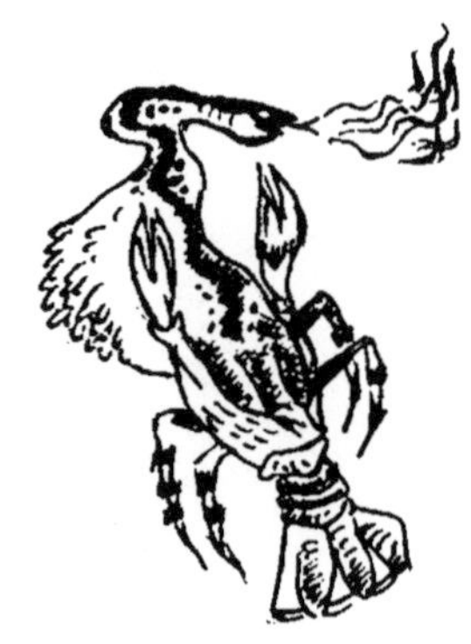

Disobedience speaks:

"Why should someone like me respect the orders of others? We would lose our individuality and eccentricity if we all acted the same. We are special fellows; by nature we are unique philosophers. We are smarter and cleverer than are others. We have studied with many different gurus and know the confusion of their contradicting theories. What nonsense to listen to all this rubbish. Nature is alien to us; so that even if we could understand the song of the birds or the message of the flowers, we would not be more intelligent. Only our own will and our own lifestyles are useful. And that's what makes us happy and prosperous. We can do only what we understand. Everything else is to our disadvantage. What counts is what we can see and hold in our hands. Therefore, we judge everything; is it useful and does it give us profit? This is in accordance with the will of God when he said: 'Let man have dominion over all the earth.' God has submitted everything to us so we could have the benefit" (LVM).

Healing Words of Obedience

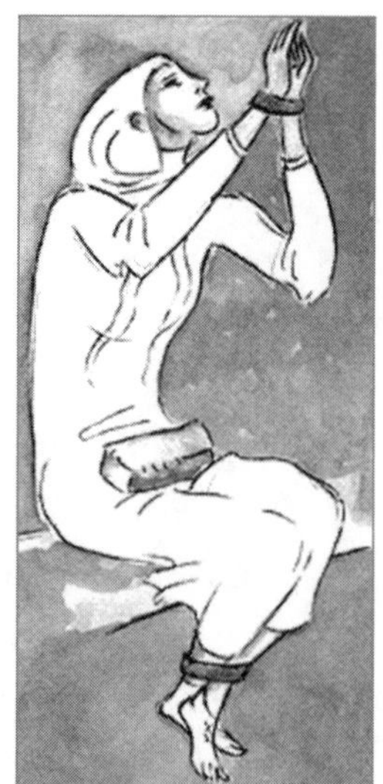

Obedience, the core of the will of God, answers:

"I follow God and therefore enjoy his strong support. I am the eye of God and was there, when the universe was created with the powerful words "Let there be light." From the beginning the angel of disobedience fights against me, but without success—for I am the sun, the moon, and the stars; I am in the roar of springwater. I am the root of all God's works. I am like the soul in the body. I am God's will and his operator; I do what God wants me to do. I was there from the very beginning and God has created everything with me. I am God's instrument, God's law, and God's original blessing (LVM).

Organ Relationship

Disobedience, defiance, disregard, resistance, fighting back, and insolence relate to the pathology of the nervous system in the region of vertebrae Th12. This area regulates the visceral organs—the kidneys, liver, and pancreas—as well as the gastrointestinal system, the back, the legs, and the urogenital organs.

Hildegard describes in her vision a restless person living in darkness and dancing on a hot plate (restless-legs syndrome). Little worms are snapping, causing inflammation and infection such as vasculitis, phlebitis, and erysipelas (LVM).

Spiritual risk factors—disobedience and defiance, for example—can give rise to autoaggressive diseases like gastritis, colitis, hepatitis, and nephritis, along with sexual disorders.

Spiritual Healing

Spiritual healing of disobedience, defiance, and rebellion needs the healing power of obedience. We learn obedience if we live for a certain period alone. After a short time in isolation, we are happy and thankful for any company, even that of people we did not respect before. Disobedient people should fast and strengthen the body with physical fitness and sauna in combination with brush massage.

Reading and praying Psalm 119:57–64, John 14:23–24, and I Peter 1:13–15 can aid us on the path to true obedience.

20. *Infidelitas*	*Fides*
Lack of faith	**Faith**
Infidelity	Fidelity, confidence
Distrust	Trust
Doubt	Certainty
Disloyalty	Loyalty
Skepticism	Reliance

Crystal Therapy

The sapphire increases spiritual wisdom, trust, and faith.

Have the sapphire set in gold, then wear it on a chain and lick it several times a day.

Faith is the absolute trust in God and Creation, summarized in the words of the Nicene Creed: "I believe in the one God, Creator of heaven and earth, and of all things visible and invisible." Faith does not mean belief in uncertainty; it means belief in the wisdom of God, which all of us can experience during our lifetime. Faith has a lot to do with knowledge, the knowledge of nature and of the laws of nature.

According to Hildegard, all science comes from God. It is the knowledge of life from the fruits of the tree of life. It is not the fruits from the tree of the knowledge of good and evil; those are the fruits of mankind and the fruits of infidelity. The fruits from the tree of life are different. They have no side effects and cause no damage; their only purpose is to support life and sustain it.

FAITH: A MIRROR OF GOD

Faith reflects the power of God in all aspects of our daily lives. Nutrition, food and drink, clothing, the houses we live in, our lifestyles, our cultural lives—all are a reflection of God. Everything we accomplish should sustain and support life.

But, as everybody knows, just the opposite is true. Profiteering has turned Western society into a global hospital. More than 80 percent of the population suffers and dies because of a stressful lifestyle and harmful nutrition. Only

10 percent of all sicknesses are caused by environment or genes. Money-oriented, high-tech medicine wants us to believe most diseases are genetic—"one gene, one disease—in order to make a profit from the new genetic exchange medicine. But every clear-minded person knows even the best DNA can be destroyed by lifestyle and inappropriate nutrition. In addition, technology manipulates food, water, clothing, and houses. We are sick from the "sick-house" syndrome, food allergies, chemicals in everything we touch and smell. We grill the universe with satellites and microwave our food to carcinogenic poison.

Faith and trust are key factors in protection from this global plague. It is our original purpose to sustain life and creation with natural fruits from the tree of life. These fruits are found in the six works of compassion, which are the foundation for health and wellness. "I was hungry and you gave me food, I was thirsty and you gave me drink, I was a stranger and you welcomed me, I was naked and you clothed me, I was sick and you visited me, I was in prison and you came to me" (Matthew 25:35–36).

Jesus encourages man to venture into the future with his message: "I am the way, the truth, and the life." For this one needs faith. Infidelity creates a negative world and a blocking effect for getting well. Infidelity has a dismal gloom covered with black eyes where its head should be.

Harmful Words of Lack of Faith

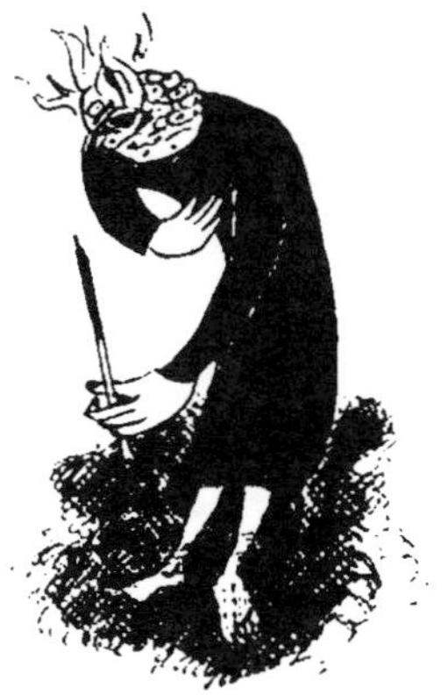

Lack of Faith speaks:

"I know no other life than this one here that I can see, feel, and understand. What do I care about eternal life? I find no reality other than that which I see here. I want to go my way and do my thing, exactly as I know and understand. Even if I were to investigate the sun and moon, I would not find an answer for my life. Therefore, I want to do only that which brings me profit" (LVM).

Healing Words of Faith

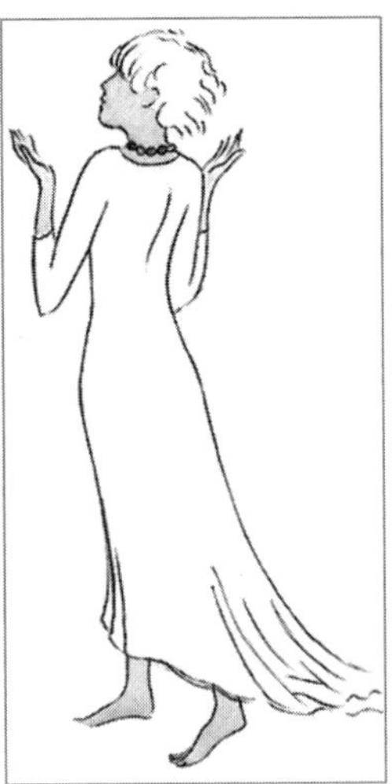

Faith responds:

"Oh, you terrible Lack of Faith, you turn everything upside down into its opposite. You have an urge to damage and cause destruction if that would bring you profit or an advantage. You cannot see the way to salvation and health, because your eyes are darkened. You are damned and lost, because you hide from the light and beauty of faith.

"I praise God with the angels and trust God, and I want what God wants. I judge and make all my decisions in harmony and in accordance with the prophets, scribes, and wise men. I am a mirror of God and reflect all aspects of life, radiating brightly the laws of God" (LVM).

What Is Faith?

Faith is the belief in life and in life energy.

> I am faith and I believe there is one God in three persons of one essence and of equal glory, one God to be worshiped. Therefore, I will have faith and trust in the Word (Proverbs 3:5), and I will not blot out God's name (Revelation 3:5) from my heart for all eternity" (SC III, vision 8:5).

Who is God? In the words of the Nicene Creed, "I believe in the one God, Creator of heaven and earth, and of all things visible and invisible." God created the visible, material, and the invisible spiritual worlds, which are part of every human nature.

Who is the Christ? According to the Nicene Creed, "Christ was fully God, one God from God, one essence, one substance with God without division, without separation, but nevertheless fully human with a physical and spiritual body" (I Corinthians 15:44).

He is the one through whom humanity is bonded to divinity for all times. The concept of salvation includes "health and wholeness" for body and soul—in modern words, nutrition and the art of living as well as awareness of the whole creation. The greatest ideas today are of freedom and liberation, liberation of all men and women from whatever binds them, both internally and externally, even their bonds to the political illnesses of our times.

In practice, faith in Christ empowers people to join in solidarity with the poor and oppressed and to honor a commitment to change social injustice and the errors of the world. Salvation has to do with the well-being of the whole creation. A vision from Hildegard shows the human hanging in the graphic net of the entire universe embraced by the love of Christ and God. And she means all humans of the globe—Christians, Muslims, Jews, Buddhists, Hindus, believers, and nonbelievers.

Who is the Holy Spirit? According to the Nicene Creed, the spirit is "the giver of life" of the cosmos, of creation, and of human life. The Hebrew word *ruach,* the breath of life, means "spirit," "breath," and "wind" all at the same time. Nowadays we would ask, What difference does the spirit make? The giver of life gives us power to work for natural medicine, freedom, peace, and a culture that respects the dignity of every human and of creation. Believing and doing go hand in hand. What difference does faith make? It helps us to love the world and all the people in it. Any other spirit who destroys life comes from disrespect for and lack of faith in God's world and kills life for profit and possession.

Organ Relationship

Lack of Faith relates to the pathology of the nervous system in the region of the vertebrae L1 to the lumbar region of L3, especially L1. The nerve L1 controls the iliac muscle; the muscles of the hips, thighs, and legs; the lumbar plexus; the buttocks; and the arteries and veins of the legs and knees. This area is also responsible for the weakening of the female and male sex organs.

Hildegard sees in her vision of Lack of Faith a stinking manure pile with worms, gas, and foul odor. This condition is a symbol of symptoms caused by leaky-gut syndrome. Millions of allergens, bacteria, viruses, and yeasts penetrate through the holes of the intestines into the bloodstream. These invaders stimulate so many weapons in our immune systems that autoaggression ultimately destroys the whole body. Autoaggression and inflammation of these organs, like nephritis and colitis, and sexual disorders can be caused by the spiritual risk factors of too much disrespect and a thirst for fame.

Spiritual Healing

The state of fidelity and trust can be reached through fasting and by strengthening our body with fitness and sauna in combination with brush massage before we shower and exercise. If we practice faith and trust daily, we will never need to look anywhere else.

Daily prayers (like Psalms 91, 118, and 119:73–80) and rituals can strengthen our faith in God and teach us to keep our eyes wide open for the gifts from the universe, which are already within us.

21. *Desperatio* **Despair**	*Spes* **Hope**
Desperation, anxiety	Confidence
Pessimism	Optimism
Depression	Being uplifted
Heartache, sorrow	Assurance
Lack of faith	Conviction

Crystal Therapy

The ruby is helpful for migraines, gallbladder complaints, and other desperate conditions.

A ruby acts as a painkiller, penetrating the body when it is placed on pain centers. Remove when the pain stops.

Hope is the power to overcome a situation of despair. Hope is the result of our life experiences teaching us that after the darkness comes the light. Our experiences in the valley of tears and sorrows open the door to happiness and salvation. Life is a rhythm of day and night; the negative path leads in the direction of the positive path. Hope is the spiritual force within ourselves that no matter what happens, even the worst possible scenario, we are always in God's hands.

Despair and hopelessness are the result of infidelity and trust in the things of the visible world. As soon as the material world crashes, there is nothing to grasp.

In Hildegard's vision, Despair looks like an exceptional woman dressed in black clothes. Despair appears as a veiled form with arms pressed tightly on her breast. Sulfuric mountains burn and fall in the foreground and a horrible thunderstorm rages in the background.

Harmful Words of Despair

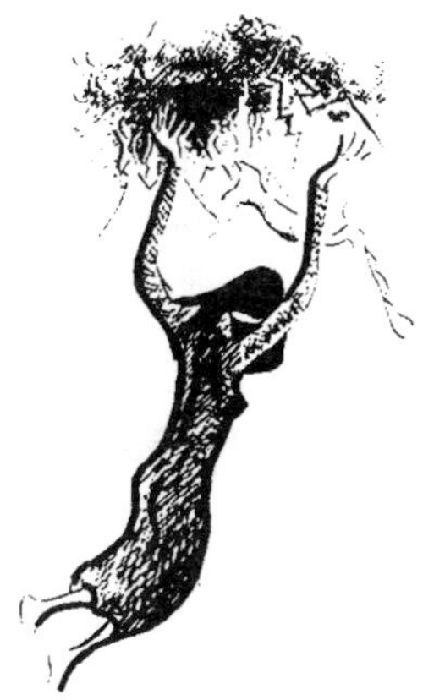

Despair laments:

"I am shocked and desperate; who can comfort me? Who can rescue me from this catastrophe that is crushing me? The fire of hell is blazing around me and God's zeal has thrown me into the jaws of hell. What is left for me if not death? I no longer find joy or comfort in sinning. There is nothing good in the whole world" (LVM)!

We all know the infectious disease of hopelessness and desperation, which can pollute the entire environment. Some people are pessimistic and depressive by nature; everything is black because they are melancholic and see everything from its worst side. Pessimism attracts pessimism and the fear of sickness attracts sickness. Hopelessness kills the immune system.

The careless diagnosis of a physician—"You have an incurable disease" or "You are a hopeless case"—blocks every possibility of getting well again unless you have trust in God. Hope is the strongest healing power. It can lift up the healing forces within us and mobilize the real spiritual power of the universe so much that the "hopeless case" becomes a rock in the ocean and helps others. Nothing is incurable and there is no hopeless case in

Hildegard's medicine unless you block yourself from healing. There is always something you can do: eat healthy food or cultivate an optimistic approach, for example. Even when we die, we are born to a new life without pain and desperation.

Hope is the power of God within us that makes the impossible possible and brings about an abundance of fruits from little things like a seed in the ground. Hope fights despair.

Healing Words of Hope

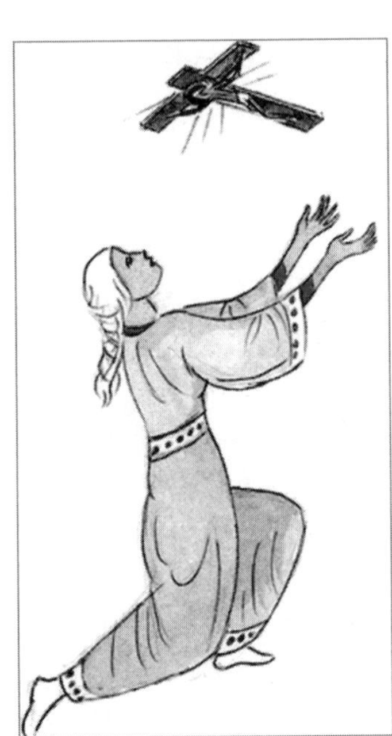

Hope answers:

"O Despair, you are the hotbed of sickness and food for Satan. You don't know and you don't have any idea what good is in God. Nobody can help you if you search for salvation in the outside world. True help for your inner void comes only from the power of God you have within yourself. Even the bad coming from God helps us to see the good. God created heaven and earth and all energy comes from him; even hell is under his control. All reward comes from him alone and every judgment of evil proceeds from him.

"Why, therefore, do you destroy yourself when you have not even been judged yet? God is the ultimate force and no good work goes without reward. I, Hope, live close to the realm of God, nourishing all God's works and making the invisible visible. If you, Despair, always concentrate on hopelessness, sorrow, and anxiety, you will cause the worst possible situation" (LVM).

Hildegard writes:

> I am Hope. O holy God, spare those who sin. You did not forsake those who had been exiled; you elevated them on your shoulders. Do not let us perish now, because we have hope in you. (SC III, vision 8:6)

Organ Relationship

Despair, hopelessness, pessimism, depression, and desperation relate to the pathology of the nervous system in the region of L2. This area controls the intestines, especially the colon and rectum, the visceral organs, and the urogenital organs. (See Frank H. Netter, *Atlas of Human Anatomy,* plate 153, page 45.)

The nerve L2 controls the iliac muscle; the muscles of the hips, thighs, and legs; the lumbar plexus; the buttocks; and the arteries and veins of the legs and knees. This area is also responsible for stimulating the female and male sex organs.

In her vision of Despair, Hildegard sees a medical metaphor relating to intestinal disorder and dysbacteria including inflammation such as urinary infection, cystitis, and phlebitis. She describes the gastrointestinal tract as being a large and deep canal, burning with fire and stinking gas. Desperate people live in the dark because they have given up all hope of healing. The same condition is a metaphor for the symptoms caused by leaky-gut syndrome as described above in the state of lack of faith.

Spiritual Healing

Spiritual healing of despair, pessimism, and depression can be found in times of prayer, meditation, and contemplation in nature, which will eventually lead to hope, confidence, and trust. Fasting and physical exercise are not advised in order to avoid heart pain, a side effect for desolate people.

Daily prayers (Psalms 42, 56, and 130; Proverbs 3:5–6; Isaiah 25:1–9 and 40:31; and John 14:1) and rituals can strengthen our trust in God and increase the chances of recovering from a bout with despair.

22. *Luxuria*	*Castitas*
Obscenity	**Chastity**
Sex without love	Sex with love and caring
Voluptuousness	Purity
Overabundance, excess	Simplicity
Superfluity	Back to the basics

Crystal Therapy

Making sapphire wine is a ritual to follow in cases of sexual harassment and extramarital affairs.

Any person suffering from these problems should pour wine over a sapphire three times while repeating the following prayer: "I pour this wine with its powerful energy over this sapphire so that the burning passion is taken away, just like God has taken away the powers and splendor of the arrogant angel." Offer this wine and drink it together as a help in delicate situations. Sapphire wine cools sexual passion and tranquilizes the nerves.

Human sexuality is one aspect of physical activity and a part of God's divine creation. Hildegard describes this force of human nature as *amor caritatis*—erotic and mutual respect directly related to the divine life force *viriditas,* the power of green. "The human body is green," she writes, "green is the blood, a man awakens through the green power of sexuality, *viriditas* flourishes in the beauty of a woman." Love (sexual energy) is directly linked to the most beautiful force that creates life and other human beings. Sexuality transports life energy throughout the body in order to balance the humors and heal every part of us.

Hildegard describes in her medical book *Causae et Curae* how Adam noticed a strong sexual impulse during his sleep. Therefore, God created woman to give Adam's love a spiritual direction. The man became the delight of the woman and the woman the human form for his love. As soon as Adam was created, sexual energy became activated in Adam's body in order to create more life and other human beings for God's kingdom. Wisdom and happiness were aroused in Adam when he admired his wife, the mother of future generations. Eve was thrilled to see the heaven in the eyes of her husband. Mutual love between man and woman is the greatest power for ultimate fulfillment. The sexual power in a man is like a burning forest fire that can hardly be stopped, whereas the sexual arousal of a woman is easily extinguished. Female sexual energy is like sunshine, which brings up fruits and flowers.

Love is a three-dimensional process empowered through the energy of God, the Son, and the Holy Spirit. One force stimulates the nerve system and pushes the sexual fire toward the endocrine glands and the sex organs. Another force activates the bloodstream to erect the stem for the sexual act, and a third power flushes immediately after the climax an orgasmic rush with precious sexual energy in order to vitalize the entire body with happiness and satisfaction. The orgasmic rush has its origin and highest excitement in the human sex organs, just like wine coming from a wine barrel.

In accordance with worldwide spiritual wisdom and teaching, Hildegard recommends sexuality be practiced with love and discipline. Sexuality without discretion reduces the life force. However, there is nothing wrong with human sexuality as long as it is practiced with mutual love. Sexuality without love, using the genitals in a one-dimensional way, downgrades sexuality to sex and perversion.

Obscenity and sex without love as well as many other forms of perversion result from despair and hopelessness. Obscenity and luxury have the figure of a woman lying on her back. Out of her mouth comes bad smelling breath and poisonous spit. A young dog sucks on one of her breasts, a snake on the other. Whoever comes near her will be dried up like grass into hay. Sexuality, God's most beautiful life force, is degraded to obscenity.

Harmful Words of Obscenity

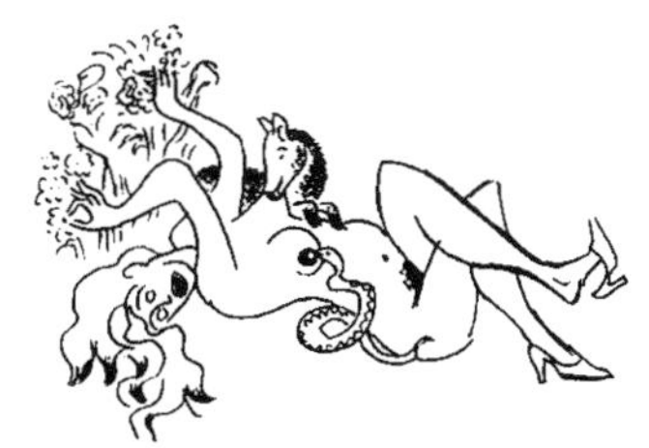

Obscenity speaks:

"Man and woman, the mirror of God's image, I will calmly drag through filth, even if it annoys the lord God. I can hurt every creature through the misuse of sexuality. I can destroy life energy and vitality when sexual energy flows into obscenity. In principle, I can captivate everybody with the desire for sexuality because that has been a part of my nature since I was born. Why should I live a simple, modest life and give up my luxurious life with extravagant glamour and sexy dances? I would become frustrated and angry or sad if I could not live according to my lust and desire. If sex and obscenity offend God, why didn't he create another world? God himself created sex appeal and sensual pleasure for quick satisfaction" (LVM).

Healing Words of Chastity

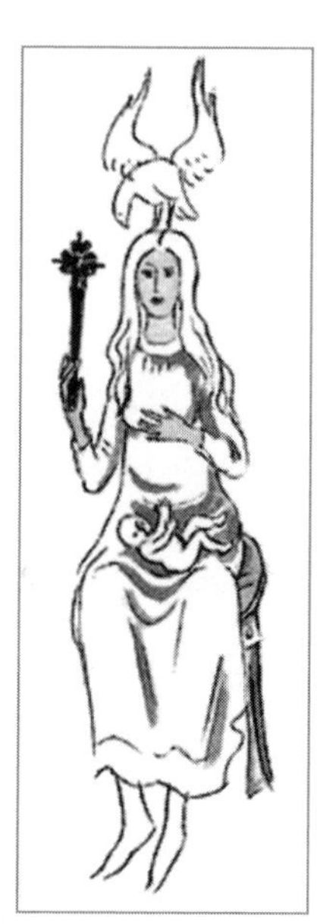

Chastity answers:

"I'm free and don't hang around in all this nasty filth and perversion. I scorn you, for you are an extravagant playboy. I don't like to be ruined by loitering. I don't use the dirty language of pornography to drag down sexuality to the gutter level.

"All my longing and desire are for the most marvelous love that actually sustains life and other human beings. I sit in the sunshine and admire the king of kings. I do this out of love of God. I am a symphony of life and enjoy the music coming from harmonious respect and compassion for others.

"I will not permit this beautiful creation to be destroyed or made dirty and ugly through sexual offense or the filth of obscenity. Heaven and earth throw us into confusion because you, Obscenity, have nothing to do with love. I have a normal relationship with God and God is love" (LVM).

If you have God, you have love, and your sexuality is the most natural fulfillment of genuine love. The devil hates love and pure sexuality.

> I am Chastity. I am free and not bound. I have passed through the purest of fountains, the purest and the most loving Word of God. I passed through the Word and went out from the Word. I trample underfoot the very proud and the devil, who are not strong enough to bind me. The devil has been cut off from me because I wish to live naturally in the love of God. (SC III, vision 8:7)

Organ Relationship

Obscenity, voluptuousness, overabundance, excess, and superfluity relate to the pathology of the nervous system in the region of vertebra L3. This area controls the descending colon, rectum, and the urogenital organs: the external genitalia, prostate, uterus, and ovaries. (See Frank H. Netter, *Atlas of Human Anatomy,* plate 153, page 45.)

The genitor-femoral nerve L3 controls the iliac muscle; the muscles of the hips, thighs, and legs; the lumbar plexus; the buttocks; and the arteries and veins of the legs and knees. This area is responsible for the strength of the female and male sex organs.

In her vision of obscenity and luxury, Hildegard sees different forms of sexual perversions. Each has different physical consequences.

People going through adultery and divorce feel like scapegoats and suffer from low resistance to fever and pain. Both partners lose all their power and strength; divorce is a bit like dying. The power of life is weakened, and life span may be cut short.

People living in unnatural love destroy the natural human image and have to consider the consequences of a destroyed immune system (AIDS). Hildegard describes infectious diseases related to filth and shit as burning like hot water.

Sodomy turns people into animals being beaten in a pigsty. Their sicknesses hurt like burning thorns and needles (LVM).

Spiritual Healing

Spiritual healing of obscenity, voluptuousness, and excess occurs during intensive fasting and physical exercise. In addition to the hard treatment, Hildegard recommends coarse clothing and physical fitness with cold water and brush massage.

Simplify your life in every respect and avoid wasting it in obscenity.

Daily prayers (like Psalms 19, 24:3–4 and 51, and 119:9; Matthew 5:8; Philippians 4:8–9; I Timothy 5:22; Hebrews 13:4; and I John 3:1–3) and rituals can strengthen our love of God and increase the chances of recovery after a stage of sexual perversion.

Chapter 6

THE SOUTHMAN

In chapter 4 Hildegard sees the cosmic man overlooking the south and west. The earth on which the man stands from his knees to his calves is rich in life energy *(viriditas)* and humors and brings forth blossoms and fruits (adornment) for the prime of life. These virtues show us the work of God on man, as in the incarnation of Jesus, the Son of God and man. The anatomical significance of this region (knees to calves) relates to sexuality, fertility, and vitality. Hildegard describes eight traditional virtues representing the moral force in the world after the death of Jesus. Everyone in contact with the message of Christ can embody these virtues and enrich his character, thus ascending to the same wisdom of Christ. But the old eight vices or imperfections must die, as they destroy life energy.

23.	*Injustitia* (injustice)	*Justitia* (justice)
24.	*Torpor* (lethargy)	*Fortitudo* (fortitude)
25.	*Oblivio* (oblivion)	*Sanctitas* (holiness)
26.	*Inconstantia* (instability)	*Constantia* (stability)
27.	*Cura terrenorum* (concern for worldly goods)	*Caeleste desiderium* (heavenly desire)
28.	*Obstinatio* (obstinacy)	*Compunctio cordis* (remorse)

29.	*Cupiditas* (craving)	*Contemptus mundi* (letting go)
30.	*Discordia* (discord)	*Concordia* (concord)

23.	***Injustitia***	***Justitia***
	Injustice	**Justice**
	Unfairness	Fairness
	Immorality	Decency
	Crookedness	Integrity
	Dishonesty	Honesty
	Wickedness	Righteousness

Crystal Therapy

The peridot or olivine is the stone of wisdom.

Wear a necklace with peridot and "this stone will strengthen the intellect and wisdom as well as creativity," writes Hildegard. "Enlightenment and good knowledge will never disappear when you wear the peridot on your heart." The "wisdom chain" will help you to keep your peace of mind during times of injustice.

The House of Wisdom

Justice, fortitude, and holiness live in partnership in the house of wisdom. These forces bring each child into the reality of the world of adults. Life provides us many opportunities to gain wisdom. Wisdom is the result of life experiences and has nothing to do with intelligence or education. It is almost impossible to teach wisdom. Sometimes it's genetic; sometimes it's a result of going through many life crises. In every respect, wisdom is the ability to be confident, knowing that behind all evil and frustration is something good. Sense is hiding behind all nonsense, and every enemy is a potential friend.

Injustice, weakness, and oblivion can lead to justice, fortitude, and holiness. Wisdom is following a spiritual path. The power of righteousness, strength, and holiness is holding the universe together. Each is a prime force that rules our lives. Injustice, weakness, and drinking and eating in oblivion (complete forgetfulness) are the enemies that destroy them.

"Do not worry about your life, what you will eat or drink, or what you will wear. But seek first his kingdom and his righteousness, and all these things will be given to you as well" (Matthew 6:25–33).

The pig, who is always eating, is the symbol of Injustice. It has a deer head and a bear tail, and the rest of the body looks like that of a pig because Injustice goes down in the mud. Injustice is the feeling of being superior, of being bigger and better than the rest of the world.

Harmful Words of Injustice

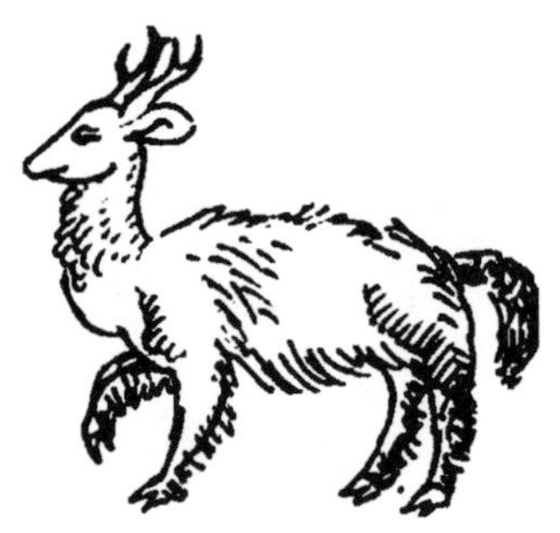

Injustice speaks:

"Do I care about justice? No way! I want to be not a creature of God, but rather a lazy donkey that needs the whip to respect others. But I'm smarter than all others. I know how I can benefit from the power of the sun, the moon, the stars, and all other creatures. Why should I limit myself in regard to the others? My place is bigger if I put down everyone else. My knowledge and know-how are more advanced than anybody else's; therefore, I use it to my advantage and exploit the rest of the world" (LVM).

There is no injustice in the universe—everybody has his place and everything has its meaning. Justice and fairness are like an orchestra, in that everybody plays together. Justice has respect and recognizes the dignity of all humankind, in whom heaven and earth come together.

Healing Words of Justice

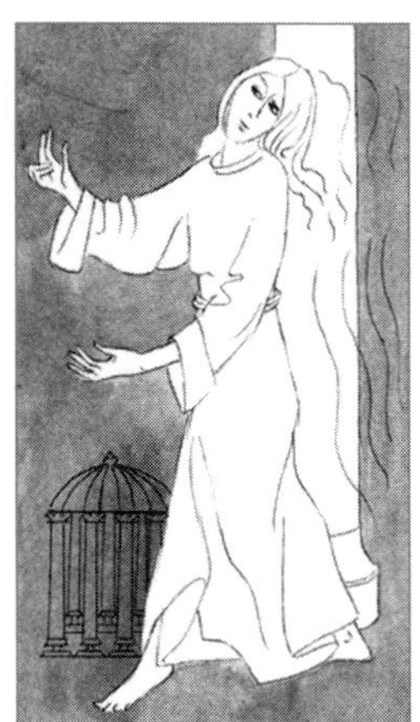

Justice responds:

"You, Injustice, are terribly in error if you look down on others. Knowledge increases when we learn from each other. You can achieve everything if you respect others and work together with nature. Why do you despise man, this incarnation of heaven and earth? Why do you reject the teachings and gifts of the Holy Spirit? Man is a temple of God in which the seven gifts of the Holy Spirit are incorporated. The seven mind-spirits rule the course of our life: wisdom, understanding, counsel, courage, knowledge, worship, and respect for God and Creation.

"I, Justice, am a symphony in which everybody can hear the harmony of God's creation. Justice is the crown jewel of creation. I respect creation, from which I acquire great knowledge and the ability to harmonize with my fellow man. Everybody rejoices in me because I am the impulse for justice. No earthly force can destroy me, as I am a gift from the source of life.

"I awake with the sunrise because I am the beloved friend of God. I am the spirit coordinator and never withdraw from God. I am the inborn basis for moral stamina and generate spiritual bravery in all human beings. I am the power that causes trees to blossom that neither winter can destroy nor storms tear down. A forest fire cannot destroy my power. I am the power of all powers and nobody can defeat me" (LVM).

In the last two thousand years, Christian society has tried to battle evil in order to eradicate the devil and his satanic work against life and humans, but without success. Fights and conflicts, burning of men and women as heretics or witches, a world war against Hitler, wars against Saddam Hussein and Milocevic, atomic bombs dropped on Japan—these can destroy the brutal and cynical drama of injustice on earth. And it is a paradox that the more we fight, the stronger injustice becomes. All righteousness, strength, beauty, and holiness have been systematically destroyed by a malignant race from another dimension.

We humans can never destroy evil! We need strong divine support against it. Hildegard warned her contemporaries, including emperors, kings, and even the pope, that the Christian message is good news of love and that wars and fighting against evil, including the Crusades, would increase evil and even harm Christianity.

Now, at the beginning of a new century, there are many questions. Will we finally understand or will we continue fighting? Will we spend more money on soldiers and weapons, on lawyers and prisons, or will we learn the lessons of justice?

THE HUMAN BEING: SYNTHESIS OF HEAVEN AND EARTH

Even if you want to, you cannot eradicate evil: Evil is a part of each and every one of us. The desire to be without sin is not human and reminds us of the old desire to be "like God." We are a combination of heaven and earth, good and bad, and live in this polarity; otherwise, we would not be human. But the choice is up to us. We have the free will to choose on which side we will live. "In the knowledge of both forces," writes Hildegard, "good and evil, humans are really free. In knowing the good we love God and answer with good deeds; the same God we have to fear if we do evil."

On the whole, evil helps the good to grow. Therefore, look at evil and see the positive message behind it. Hildegard compares us to an eagle: "Look up to the eagle. As soon as one wing is injured, he cannot fly and has to stay on earth. In the same way, we humans fly with two wings according to our free will. The right wing symbolizes knowing the good, the left wing knowing the evil. Knowing evil has to serve knowing good. Evil makes us strong and wise and just. Remember that you are born that way and cannot be without evil."

Look for blessings from your friends, the angels who show us the way for our spiritual activity. The power of God's justice is inexhaustible if you stay on his side and accept the friendship of angels, the main sponsors of justice.

> We, the angels of justice, are heavenly soldiers ready to fight against evil and overcome the devil's wickedness and worthlessness. Otherwise, people will not be be saved from the adversity of the devil. And just as the devil tried to fight against divinity in the beginning of time, the Antichrist will try to resist the incarnation of the Word in the latest of times. Lucifer fell in the beginning of time. But we virtues have been placed to fight against the cunning and bragging of the devil, who swallows up souls with his trickery. All the craftiness of the devil leads to nothing in the souls of the just, for the devil is confused by so many different directions. God is known through us, not hidden but instead made manifest, because God is just in all his ways. (SC III, vision 9:2)

Organ Relationship

Injustice, unfairness, immorality, and wickedness relate to the pathology of the nervous system in the region of the vertebra L4. This area controls the descending colon, the rectum, and the urogenital organs—especially the external genitalia, prostate, uterus, and ovaries. (See Frank H. Netter, *Atlas of Human Anatomy,* plate 153, page 45)

The genitor-femoral nerve L4 also controls the iliac muscle and the muscles of the hips, thighs, and legs; the lumbar plexus; the buttocks; and the arteries and veins of the legs and knees. This area is responsible for the strength of the female and male sex organs.

In her vision Hildegard sees injustice as a result of evil spirits and manipulation, symbolically represented by demons, leading to terror, war, and disease. The demons come with fiery torture, dangerous worms that cause inflammation and violation.

The war-propaganda industry is fully aware of this influence. First of all, war is a business. In order to convince young people to kill other people, an evil enemy more or less like a satan has to come into view. Hitler, Stalin, Saddam Hussein, and Milocevic are prime examples, as they initiated chaos and hell on earth. The next step is a storm of anger motivating the nation ready to fight. The rest is tax money to pay both the weapons industry to destroy and the reconstruction industry to repair the devastation. Injustice has been the evil spirit bringing war and pain worldwide for the last two thousand years.

THE HUMAN SOUL IS A SYMPHONY

Hildegard writes:

"Attune to the flow of justice and praise the Creator in harmony. God resounds in joyful harmony with all of his creation. He uses rationality and the creative arts to establish harmony and justice in his creation. This resounds in the whole universe. In the beginning, when God created man, he gave him common sense in order to rejoice and celebrate. Praise the Lord in sweetest wisdom that all of creation can resonate in harmony and justice, because the human soul is like a symphony and has the sound of a pleasant melody. The soul is sad when she hears the heavenly symphony because she remembers her home is in heaven and she is living as a refugee in exile on earth" (LVM).

Spiritual Healing

Spiritual healing of injustice needs the spirit of justice, which is a gift that comes from intense fasting and physical exercise. Hildegard recommends wearing coarse clothing and practicing physical fitness with cold water and brush massage.

Daily prayers with the words of Psalms 1:1–3, 19:7–14, 51, 101, and 119:33–40, 41–48, 65–72, 97–104, and 105–112 and rituals can strengthen our trust that justice lies only in God. The entire universe is based on the law of justice: "What you do good or evil comes back to you, good or evil."

24. *Torpor*	*Fortitudo*
Lethargy	**Fortitude**
Habitual idleness, listlessness	Fearlessness
Loafing, inactivity	Determination
Weakness, sluggishness	Stamina
Laziness	Moral strength

Stupor, dullness	Bravery
Apathy, passivity	Steadfastness

Crystal Therapy

The emerald is useful for every weakness, including lethargy. It restores moral strength and steadfastness.

Wear an emerald as a ring or necklace and use as a pain remover by placing it on the irritated spot. For severe pain attacks, place the emerald in your mouth several times a day.

Fortitude is strong like a rock in the ocean; nothing can disturb it. Fortitude is the power to swim against the current. God supplies fortitude with weapons from the divine army, a helmet with strong life energy, a compass to find the right way, and a sword, the symbol for God's Word, to separate good from evil. Fortitude is as strong as steel and fights together with righteousness and holiness against cowardice and lethargy.

Lethargy, with a childish face under white hair, wears a faded shirt with which he tries to cover his feet and other body parts. Lethargy looks like a shapeless bag of flour.

Harmful Words of Lethargy

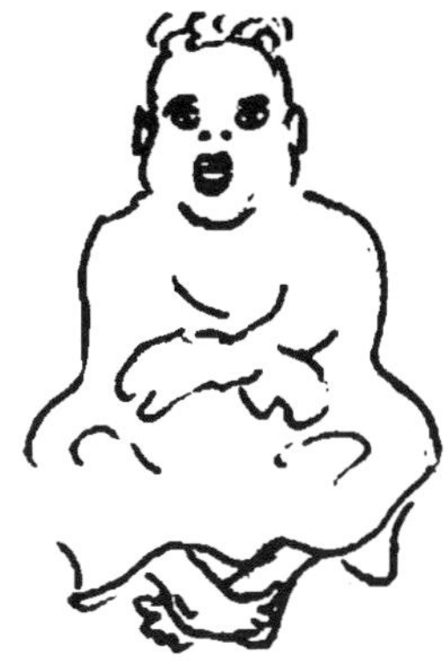

In a daze, as if intoxicated, this second character speaks:

"Why should I accept such a dull, hard life? Why should I have pains and trouble? Everybody can do what he wants according to his ego in self-fulfillment. Everything is a waste of effort. Work is a waste of time. I find a better life than the others do in comfort and in my aversion for work. Work just does not suit me. Even if I avoid hardships and other dangers, why would God let me perish for that reason" (LVM)?

Lethargy and irresponsibility are brothers and sisters. More and more people refuse to take responsibility for themselves and for others. Typical of this is the fear of making decisions and the reluctance to get married and establish a family. Many people refuse to work for their own living and expect others to support them. Fortitude and strength conquer lethargy and weakness.

Healing Words of Fortitude

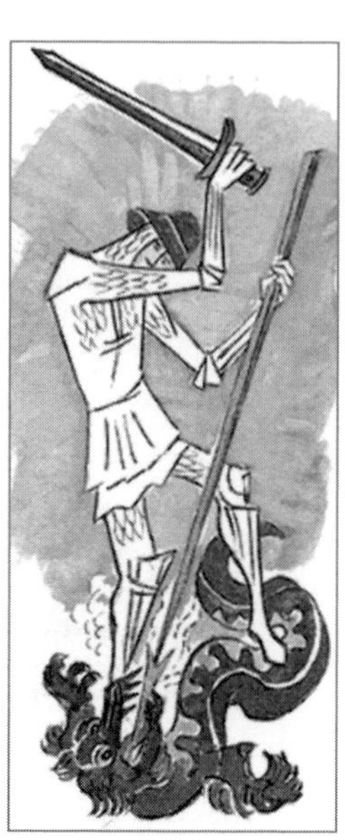

Hildegard describes the health-promoting power of Fortitude:

"I, Fortitude, tell you, Lethargy, you are dust from dust! You were useless from the beginning, a monstrous freak. You are not even equal to the worm, who at least takes the trouble to dig for his food in the ground, nor to the birds, who build nests and care for their babies. What is life but pain and labor? This life is far from the land of milk and honey. You, bastard of weakness, are excluded from divine wisdom, as you are looking for that which nobody can give: happiness without effort.

"I am like the strong lion and work very hard for humanity in the palace of the king. I, with joyous energy and exuberance, fly over the universe to aid all people and nations who ask me for help" (LVM).

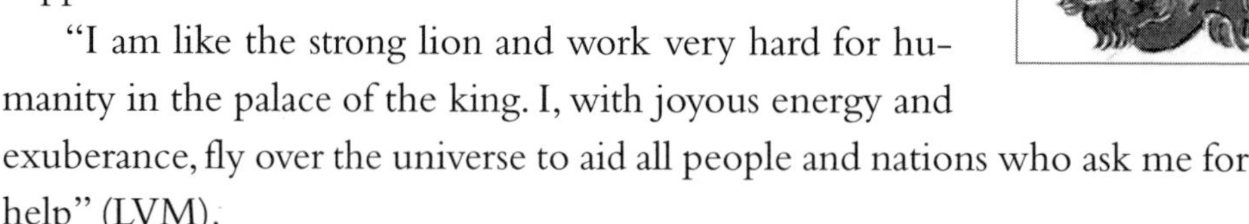

Fortitude and endurance are a divine present in times of severe trouble and desperation. All of a sudden light comes to a desperate situation and changes its hopelessness. Sometimes a person comes like an angel to encourage and comfort, when everything else looks cheerless and dark. Most of all the Word of God or a prayer can help.

> O most strong God who is able to oppose and to fight against you, Lethargy! The ancient serpent, the diabolical dragon, is not able to fight against you. Furthermore, I want to fight against this dragon with your help. That way, no one may prevail against me or hurl me down—neither the strong nor the weak, neither a leader nor one cast down, neither the noble nor the inglorious, neither the rich nor the poor. I want to be like the strongest of swords, and I want to make all weapons unconquerable and suitable for the wars of God. I want to be like the sharpest edge of a sword; no one will be able to shatter me then. I have risen up to drive out the devil through the most strong God. I also want to be a dependable

> refuge for frail people, giving a sharper edge to the softness of such people so they will be able to defend themselves. O most sweet and most pious God, help those trampled underfoot. (SC III, vision 9:3)

You will become the man on the wheel in a stormy ocean. You will find the heavenly way by looking to God and God's strength and God will provide you with all you need and deserve. You will receive physical energy and a spiritual mind, because you have the father and all you need within you.

Organ Relationship

Lethargy, weakness, cowardice, inactivity, and torpor are related to the pathology of the nervous system in the area of the vertebra L5. This region controls the descending colon, the rectum, and the urogenital organs, especially the external genitalia, prostate, uterus, and ovaries. (See Frank H. Netter, *Atlas of Human Anatomy,* plate 153, page 45). Nerve L5 also controls the iliac muscle and the muscles of the hips, thighs, and legs; the lumbar plexus; the buttocks; and the arteries and veins of the legs and knees. This area is responsible for stimulation of the female and male sex organs.

Spiritual lethargy corresponds to the different symptoms caused by an immune weakness, such as chronic fatigue, nervous breakdown, and depression. Hildegard sees in her vision of indolence different forms of lung diseases and inflammations, symbolized in a darkness void of air and filled with fire and fiery clubs that represent the various forms of chronic obstructive pulmonary disease (COPD), such as chronic bronchitis, chronic asthma, pneumonia, cystic fibrosis, and emphysema (LVM).

Meditation on Fortitude and Strength

Surprisingly, we often find fortitude and strength in people of weak physical power, sometimes in those who are crippled or handicapped in some other way. There is a long list of personalities in history who achieved miracles. It is a secret of God that he selects the weakest to reveal his miracles.

Hermanus Contractus, a monk from southern Germany, was born in 1013 with irreversible brain damage and throughout his life (he died 1054) he could not speak properly and was unable to move. He became a universal genius who founded the first university. He is the author of the first history of that time beginning with the birth of Jesus: the first *historia mundi*. He invented the first "computer," which is still used in Russia and China, and was able to measure the fixed stars with his astrolabe in order to calculate the exact dates of all sun and moon eclipses before and after his time. He connected music with mathematics and composed the famous *Salve Regina*. His wisdom can be compared to that of the British Nobel Prize laureate Stephen Hawking, who lives in a similar physical state.

Hildegard selects woman as an example of strength and courage as described by King Solomon in Proverbs 31:10–28. She writes:

"A noble wife is worth far more than rubies. Her husband has full confidence in her and lacks nothing of value. She is like a merchant ship bringing her food from afar. She provides food for her family, considers and buys a field, and plants grapevines. She sets about her work vigorously; her arms are strong for the task; she sees that her trading is profitable. She opens her arms to the poor and extends her hands to the needy. She is clothed with strength and dignity; she can laugh at the days to come. She speaks with wisdom and the teaching of kindness is on her tongue. Her children wake up and call her blessed; her husband also praises her."

Spiritual Healing

The spiritual healing of lethargy, sluggishness, and apathy occurs during fasting and physical exercise.

These daily prayers—Deuteronomy 6:4–9; Psalms 28:7–9 and 46:1, 92, and 121; Isaiah 41:9–13; and Philippians 4:13—give every day a special meaning.

25. *Oblivio*	*Sanctitas*
Oblivion	**Holiness**
Forgetfulness	Remembrance
Nothingness	Sanctity

Emptiness, void	Wholeness
Being meaningless	Hallowed, meaningful
Insignificance	Importance

Crystal Therapy

Use the gold topaz and the Gold Topaz Prayer (see page 224) to protect you from harm during daily life.

Remember, your body is the visible house of the invisible God who lives within you. The presence of God provides all the energy you will need to survive, to strengthen your immune system, and to protect you from outside damage. Healing occurs when you are attuned to the presence of God, who is the source of all life energy. Whatever you call it—being at one with God, feeling at home, being connected with the universe—as soon you have this enlightened moment, you are in the center of holiness. Any activity that centers you with God can promote holiness, healing, and wholeness, which are all the same. For some it is a hearty conversation with God, a prayer, a song, a dance, painting, poetry, gardening, swimming in the ocean, mountain climbing, or simply walking through the woods. Any of these activities can provide you with holy energy.

We all experience times of strength and times of weakness. When you move too far from the center, you lose holy energy and become empty, and life seems meaningless. This is when your immune system breaks down and diseases begin. You alone know what will help you to reconnect with the holy center.

Fasting is a universal means whereby you can find the Father and holy energy within you and reactivate the spiritual symbiosis with the angel of holiness. During fasting you make the closest connection to this center; therefore, fasting is the "king's way" to health and healing. Relax into the loving center of seraphim and cherubim, become attuned to God, and heal.

The art of healing, especially Hildegard of Bingen's medicine, is always interested in restoring wholeness and well-being. This healing art occurs normally in four dimensions simultaneously: in the realms of the body, the soul, the spirit, and the environment.

Medicine of today has forgotten this. Disease is the biggest business in the

Western world. Healing occurs mainly on the physical level. We are not even interested in holistic healing, and take quick drugs with dangerous side effects that shift the symptoms from one side to the other. The eye infection is gone but produces gastritis or some other illness. The medicine creates enough clients who are chronically ill and are always hooked on some sort of treatment. Eight hundred years ago Hildegard foresaw our modern medicine, which heals only on the physical level because all eyes are closed to holistic medicine. She even foresaw a time of total darkness, during which we all will have forgotten where we came from and where we are going. Now we have forgotten the divine within us and live in a spiritual and mental stage of forgetfulness, which she calls oblivion.

Oblivion looks like a lizard with its two front feet on a black storm cloud. It has the viewpoint of a frog and has forgotten the divine (God's holy energy) in order to live according to its own ego.

Harmful Words of Oblivion

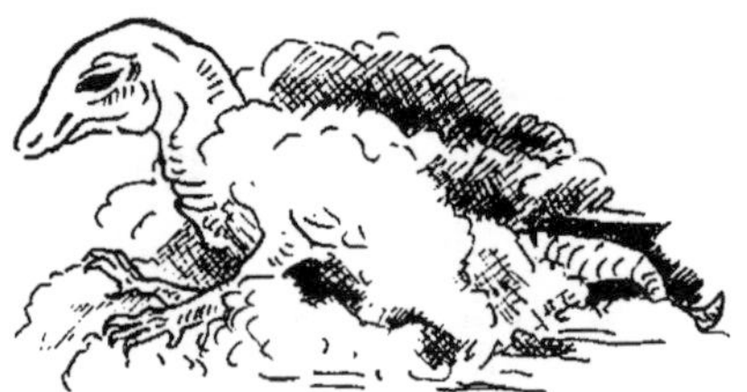

Oblivion turns everything upside down and declares that not it, but rather God, lives in forgetfulness:

"If God doesn't want to know me, and because I know nothing of him, why should I not do what I want? Besides, God doesn't want me and I'm not able to perceive or understand a thing about God. Many people tell me about eternal life, which I don't believe in, and nobody could show or prove it to me.

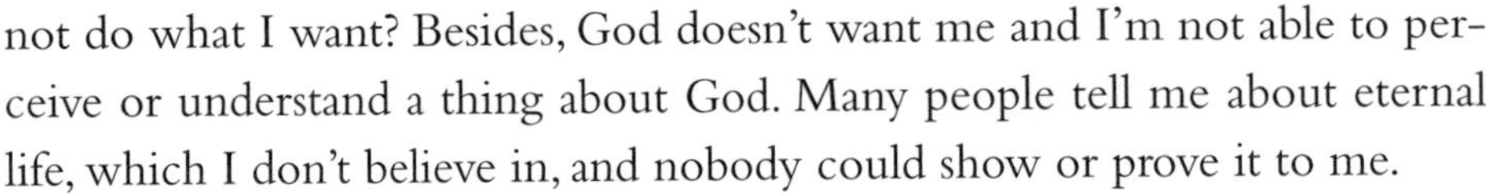

"Others show me their plans, which are of no use to me. I refuse any other gods and teachers because I pursue only my own plans.

"What I know I understand, and what I like, that is what I'll do! If there is really a God, then one thing is sure—he doesn't know me" (LVM).

When you lose your way and live in oblivion, simply remember your origin and where you are going. All the natural religions worldwide know the art of remembering. The Aborigines, the indigenous peoples of Australia, remember their origin and consider their existence of divine origin. Ninety percent of their lifetime they spent in ceremonies to remember creation based on an oral religion. Each ceremonial master had to know at least six thousand songs, dances, stories, and rituals to celebrate rites unchanged from one generation to the next. The memory of the Aboriginal masters was bigger than any computer memory of today! You can remember your own holy origin if you simply call on God and break through the void and darkness of oblivion.

Healing Words of Holiness

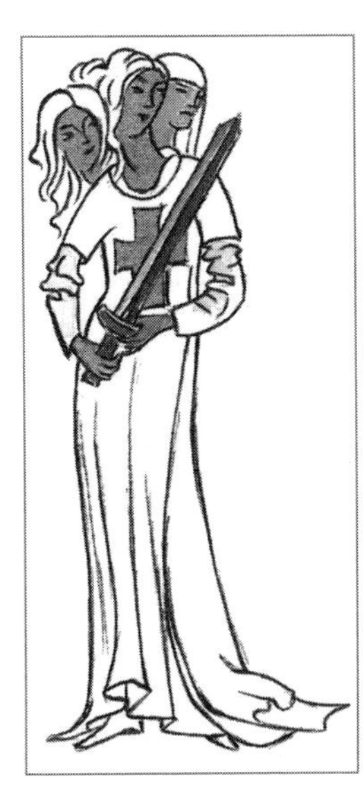

Holiness responds:

"Remember your Creator! Who gave you your life? Can't you see that only God is the origin of your life, and not yourself? Only God provides whatever you need. If you open your eyes, you will be able to see that there is more than enough of everything necessary for living, including clothing and food for everyone. Although we see everything growing, we don't know how it grows. Nobody on this earth can give life or sustain it or return death to life. Only God can do this.

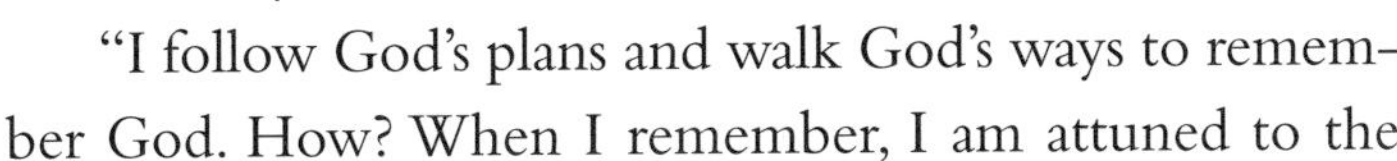

"I follow God's plans and walk God's ways to remember God. How? When I remember, I am attuned to the presence of God. I play the harp and sing, I remember and pray, and so I recognize God.

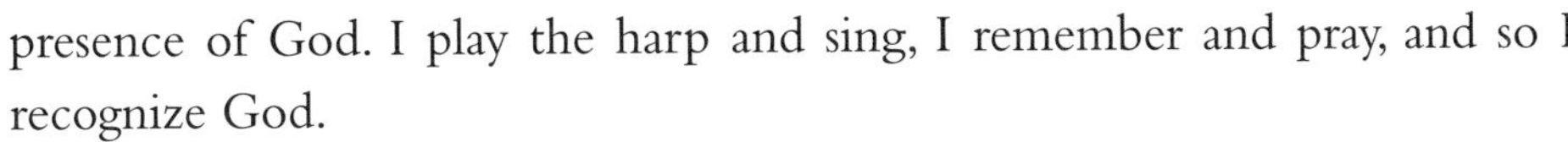

"Those who serve God and pursue his will are those who avoid evil and help others grow. I am a child of God, a leader in the divine army fulfilling God's work on earth" (LVM).

The journey toward holiness is to remind us time and again to search for ways back to God by doing God's work with modesty. The real power of holiness and healing is like love: The more you give, the more you receive. The happiest people are not those who gain a lot of money while healing, but are those who help others as God does. His name means "healer," to get well again in a holistic way. God heals like a mother—unconditionally, completely, and absolutely.

Hildegard writes:

> I rise up from holy humility. I was born from humility just as an infant is born from a mother. I was also taught and strengthened by humility just as a baby is nourished to strength through nursing. (SC III, vision 9:4)

Organ Relationship

Oblivion, forgetfulness, emptiness, insignificance, and being meaningless relate to the pathology of the nervous system in the region of the sacrum, especially S1. It is a beneficial coincidence that the virtue of holiness, healing, and wholeness relates to the spinal part of the sacrum and opens the view to the next five virtues, which live in the palace of the master of the universe Jesus Christ. The spinal nerve S1 controls the descending colon, the rectum, and the urogenital organs, especially the external genitalia and the prostate, uterus, and ovaries. (See Frank H. Netter, *Atlas of Human Anatomy,* plate 153, page 45.)

The same nerve, S1, controls the iliac muscle and the muscles of the hips, thighs, and legs; the lumbar plexus; the buttocks; and the arteries and veins of the legs and knees. This area is also responsible for the stimulation of the female and male sex organs.

In her vision of Oblivion, Hildegard sees people who can receive terrible diseases of the intestinal region, including leaky-gut syndrome, with the result being autoimmune diseases such as ulceration, nerve inflammation, and even intestinal cancer.

"I saw a deep valley with a tremendous length and depth in which a strong fire with a horrible stink was burning. Terrible worms with dreadful forms lived in this valley" (LVM).

Meditation on Healing

Healing energy flows through your body if you remember Psalm 103, which reflects the four stages of healing: adoration, atonement, healing, and rehabilitation.

Praise the Lord, O my soul;
and forget not all his benefits.
Who forgives all your sins,
and heals all your diseases,
who redeems your life from the pit,
and crowns you with love and compassion,
who satisfies your desires with good things,
so that your youth is renewed,
like the eagle.

THE POWER CENTER OF THE HUMAN SOUL

If you were able to open the sacrum from the spinal cord, you would see a power pack of spinal nerves that form the sacral plexus and the great sciatic nerve. Through these sacral nerves flows a tremendous energy from our souls to our bodies, which is responsible for the proper function of such essential organs as the intestinal tract and the sex organs, as well as the muscles, ligaments, arteries, and veins of the hips, thighs, and legs. The anatomy of the sacrum is equivalent to the power center of the human soul.

This power center provides us with an unlimited supply of energy, which we need for our survival during our journey through life. The energy from this divine source is required to sustain us through the dark side of life, through danger, difficulties, pain, and humiliation. It is given to us before we are born with the incarnation of our golden soul.

ABB SCIVIAS JESUS AND THE FIVE FORCES

Hildegard describes a magnificent palace in the city of Jerusalem, where Jesus lives in partnership with five beautiful forces. The palace symbolizes the innermost power center of the human soul. Three forces stand in front and two in back of the master of the universe. All forces begin with the letter *C*. The three forces in front are *constantia, caeleste desiderium,* and *compunctio cordis.*

Constancy gives us the ability to survive the most dangerous situations. Celestial desire is on her right and is similar to a spiritual radar necessary to find orientation in life. The force on the left side is the beating of our hearts (remorse and regret), which we need as a warning signal when we take a wrong turn. We learn to call on this power when we are alone in desperation and need the partnership of God in order to begin anew. In the back of the spiritual power station we see two lighthouses that can make extraordinary things happen. *Contemptus mundi* is the liberation force, which can free us from our addictions, obsessions, and daily enjoyable poisons; *concordia* is the power that enables us to live in harmony in a multicultural society.

All five forces are always present in this power center of the soul and will perform miracles when activated. However, a blackout may occur when we have difficulties recognizing the light within us. Power leaks may also occur through negative destructive forces such as inconstancy, worry, obstinacy, obsession, and addiction as well as disharmony. In these times we have to actively remember and find holiness to open the door to the power center of the human soul.

Spiritual Healing

Spiritual healing of forgetfulness, emptiness, and insignificance takes place during fasting and physical exercise. In addition, Hildegard recommends a retreat into the wilderness (alone) in order to find your way back to God. To do this, practice remembering where you come from and where you are going. Remember the third commandment in Exodus 20, verse 8–11: "Remember the sabbath day, to keep it holy."

This takes you to a deeper understanding of God, who lives within and connects you to the angelic forces in the universe. This newly remembered holiness opens the door to the power center of the human soul.

Read and pray Psalms 105:1–7, 106, and 111; Proverbs 3; Ecclesiastes 12:1–7; and I Corinthians 11:23–26 to grow gradually in wisdom.

26. *Inconstantia*	*Constantia*
Instability	**Stability**
Inconstancy	Constancy
Lack of character	Strength of character
Lack of personality	Strong personality
Unsteadiness	Steadiness
Unreliability	Reliability
Inconsistency	Self-control
Irresoluteness	Firmness
Hesitancy	Straightforwardness

Crystal Therapy

Jasper improves concentration and sharpens the intellect.

Place the jasper in your mouth. It will restrain a person so that he doesn't remain irresolute and inconsistent. This therapy promotes steadfastness and stability.

Stability enables us to be firm as a rock in times of heavy storms. I learned my lesson in stability during a sailboat trip in the West Indies. We were sailing in heavy seas from Martinique to the Tobago keys when suddenly, while close to the two volcanic peaks on St. Lucia, the GPS and the steering system both failed in the middle of the night. The ship was thrashing about and all members of the crew including the captain were seasick. Only Bill, an elderly skipper and the oldest man on board, had the wherewithal to go outside and maneuver the battered boat. Here and now he used the mental power of stability to find the inner strength and bravery necessary for this situation. His steadiness finally brought us forward on our journey to Tobago.

Instability is the limiting factor of power in times of darkness and disappointment. Instability is stuck tight to a wagon wheel lying in the dark. Four clubs sticking out of the wagon hit instability. The wheel turns the person around and around, symbolizing that Instability lives in a state of disruption and lack of balance. His hands are like those of an ape because all he does is silly and foolish.

Harmful Words of Instability

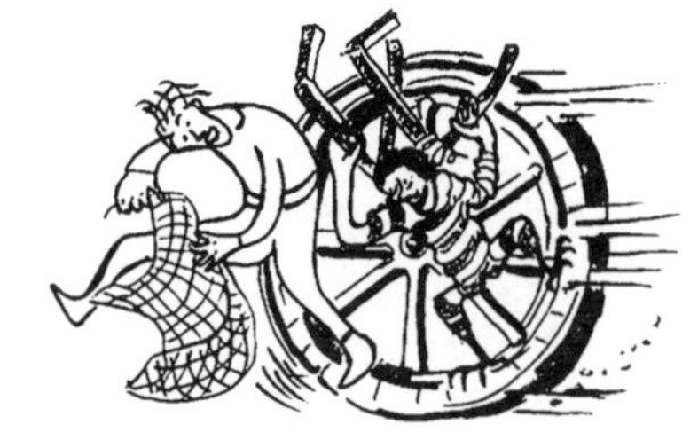

Instability believes he is cleverer and more intelligent than anybody else:

"I know exactly who I am, what I have to do, and how to do it! I like to make fools out of the wise and beggars out of the rich. I fulfill my will with every possibility. I take as much as I can from others and am not like a stupid farmer who does not harvest his fields" (LVM).

The best way to fight instability is to remember situations in your life when you received unlimited energy to overcome the difficulties.

Healing Words of Stability

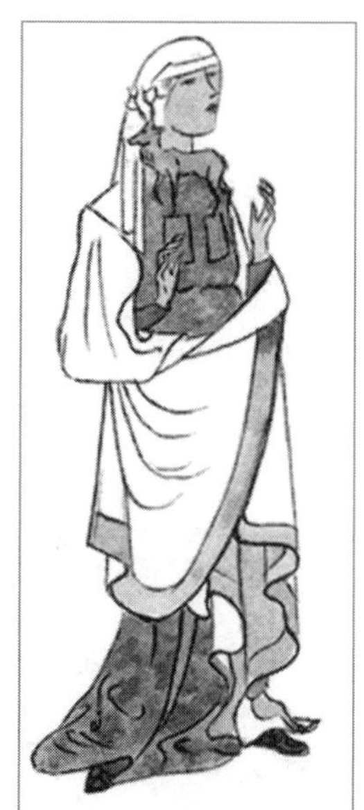

Stability responds:

"You are foolish and vain like Lucifer, who fell from heaven and crashed on earth and lost his energy. Everybody will fall in darkness and lose his energy who struggles without the divine force, as did Goliath and other demons and tyrants.

"Only God gives you the double-edged sword of clear conscience to fight evil and the club of bad conscience to foresee what is good for you. God gives you the good conscience as a ladder to climb into heaven and a bad conscience to break through and climb over difficulties. God's power is already in the deepest part of your soul.

"Why do you pursue evil and despise good? You drown in the ocean without seeing the lifeboat that could bring you to heaven" (LVM).

Stability is the fundamental power of life in moments of danger:

"I am a strong pillar and not fickle with instability. I am not stirred by a blast of the wind, as is the leaf of a tree, which is stirred by the wind and flung hither and thither. I endure by standing on true stone—that is, the true Word of God. Who is strong enough to move me? Who can injure me? Neither a strong person nor a weak one, neither a leader nor a follower, neither a rich person nor a poor one! My stability is based on the true God, who will not be moved for all eternity (Psalm 125:1). I cannot be upset because I stand on the strongest of foundations. I do not want to be among those who cry because they have been scattered about by the winds. They never remain at rest and are not stable; they are always falling to lower and lower places. I am not that way because I have been placed on a firm rock" (SC III, 10:10).

Organ Relationship

Instability, inconstancy, lack of personality, unsteadiness, unreliability, and hesitancy relate to the pathology of the nervous system in the region of the sacrum, especially S2. The spinal nerve S2 controls the descending colon, the rectum, and the urogenital organs, especially the external genitalia, the prostate, the uterus, and the ovaries. (See Frank H. Netter, *Atlas of Human Anatomy,* plate 153, page 45.)

The same nerve, S2, controls the iliac muscle and the muscles of the hips, thighs, and legs; the lumbar plexus; the buttocks; and the arteries and veins of the legs and knees. This area is responsible for invigorating the female and male sex organs.

In her vision of Instability, Hildegard sees terrible viral and bacterial diseases:

"I saw a gigantic fire with all kinds of horrible worms. People who robbed the energy of others had to burn in this fire because they did this through deceit and cunning. They were tortured by worms because of their trickery. People with instability weaken their immune system and risk the possibility of autoaggressive sicknesses, which come in many forms" (LVM).

Spiritual Healing

Spiritual healing for instability, inconstancy, and unreliability can be best accomplished by living in isolation for a time. Fasting is not recommended for unstable people because it costs too much mental energy. You can also find stability by looking for the light of the spiritual way inside yourself. Do this by awakening to your own power and experiencing the opportunity that hides behind the next obstacle.

These Bible passages are excellent for meditation:
Psalm 40, I Corinthians 15:58, and II Thessalonians 2:13–17.

Nothing is too big,
nothing too small.
The night has only twelve hours,
then comes the day.
—Bertolt Brecht

27.	***Cura terrenorum***	***Caeleste desiderium***
	Concern for worldly goods	**Heavenly desire**
	False security	Yearning for heaven
	Fear	Feeling free
	Worry	Lack of concern
	Troubles	Carefree
	Anxiety	Calm

Crystal Therapy

The amethyst is a tranquilizer and encourages self-confidence and freedom from anxiety.

All cares and worries disappear when you wear a huge amethyst ring or necklace.

Heavenly desire produces the energy to move beyond the barriers of worry into the flow of spiritual abundance. Here you will find the heavenly way, where your insecurity will be transformed into a state of peace and relaxation. Scales will fall from your eyes as you shift your attention from there and then to the here and now. You will see the rich gifts of spiritual nourishment, which you have already received in abundance. God provided you with whatever you need for this life from the moment you were born. Yearning is the spiritual radar to help you find the place within you.

Sometimes our human nature creates worries when we move too far into the daily struggle of life. The concern for worldly things makes us believe we don't have enough of what we need for our daily life. This creates anxiety and fears and an attempt to fill the inner void with material things from outside. More desire creates more pressure to work harder until we have all the money, all the things, and all the property we think we need to be happy.

But material things can never make us happy; to the contrary, at some point we begin to recognize that the possession of material objects causes loss of energy when we lose all our belongings. Only our spiritual inner gifts and values can never get lost. The power of Heavenly Desire, a partner of stability, concentrates on the purpose of life. She pushes our spiritual vision into the heavenly atmosphere, which cares that we be uplifted and filled with a flow of energy.

The concern for worldly goods drains energy from our inner power centers. Hildegard envisions Concern for Worldy Goods as a woman in a wine barrel who collects her daily possessions. Because she is a companion of instability, she has forgotten the spiritual realm. Communication and encounters with the spiritual realm do not exist in her world of daily worries. She is obsessed by "not getting enough." Her concerns and sorrows cause her hair to turn gray. Such people break under the burden of life.

Harmful Words of Concern for Worldly Goods

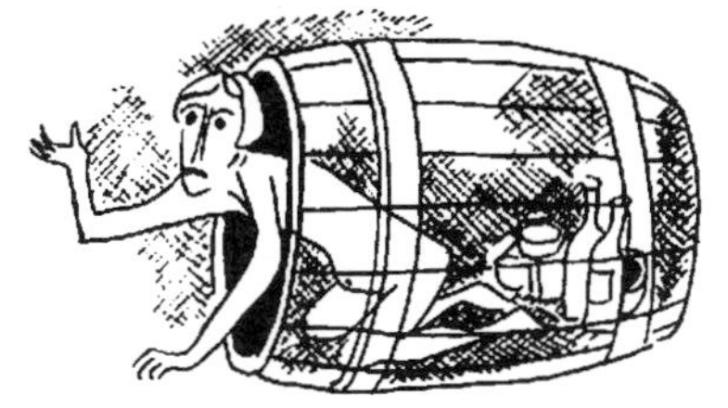

Naked, Concern for Worldly Goods stands in the dark and speaks:

"Which concern could be more important than the worries about this world? How else but with my help do grain and fruit trees grow? How but from me come grapes and all the other things that are so necessary for life? If I were to fill my eyes with tears or beat on my breast with sighs or always bend my knees, I would have nothing to eat or wear—I would live in misery! It is useless to request food from the sun, the moon, or the stars. I can survive only if I work hard to have those things I need" (LVM).

Heavenly Desire makes a clear decision to seek the loving and giving contact to God. Radiant energy will flow as soon as one is attuned to God.

Healing Words of Heavenly Desire

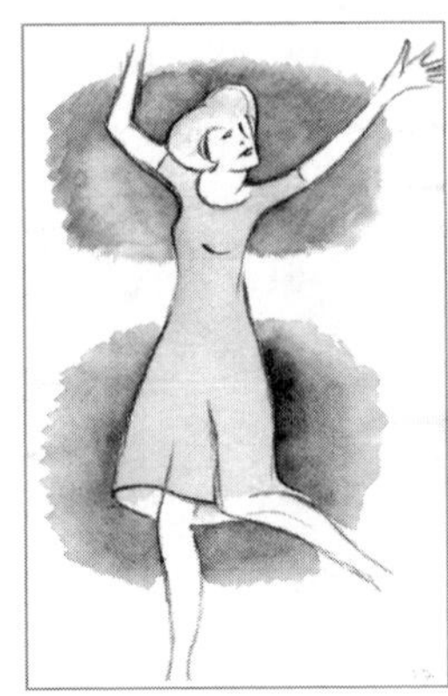

Heavenly Desire responds to Concern for Worldly Goods:

"O thief of spiritual energy, you are a hypocrite and a trickster because you have no trust in God. Don't you see that God has already given you all you need? All fruits grow through the grace of God, just as the body lives through the soul. Look at the skeleton, which decays in the earth. You cannot live without the grace of God. You achieve nothing all alone. You have completely forgotten the desire for God. What do you expect when you don't ask for help?

"Heaven is my home and I communicate with the angelic spheres to live in harmony with all creatures. For all I do and all I achieve, you are my life and the power center within me. I am a jewel among all spiritual values. I am overflowing with joy and fascinated with the loving God. I am the temple of desire for God and do everything God expects me to do. . . .

"I fly with my wings over the universe and bring eternal righteousness to earth. I see God's work face to face because I climb on top of the highest mountain, Bethel. I am searching only for holiness, joy, and happiness for the others and me. I am the abundance of harmony and the music of God's friendliness. My physical body is filled with the spiritual essence of God's love, and that is why I am both heavenly and earthly by nature" (LVM).

Yes, there is the power of the Heavenly Desire here and now in being at one with God:

"Just as a deer longs for a fountain of water, so also my soul desires you, O God" (Psalm 42:2).

> I want to leap over mountains and hills, and I want to leap over this sweet but transitory life. I want to look back to the fountain of living water, for God is full of immeasurable glory, and no one can be bored with the abundance of God's sweetness. (SC III, vision 10:11)

Organ Relationship

Concern for worldly goods, fear, worry, anxiety, trouble, and concern for the future relate to the pathology of the nervous system in the region of the sacrum, especially S3. The sacral nerve S3 controls the descending colon, the rectum, and the urogenital organs, especially the external genitalia, the prostate, the uterus, and the ovaries. (See Frank H. Netter, *Atlas of Human Anatomy,* plate 153, page 45.)

The same nerve controls the viscera and the iliac muscle, as well as the muscles of the hips, thighs, and legs; the lumbar plexus; the buttocks; and the arteries and veins of the legs and knees. This area is responsible for the stimulation of the female and male sex organs.

RICH BECOMES POOR AND POOR BECOMES RICH

In her vision of concern for the material world Hildegard sees demonic forces turning the wealth of the Western world into its greatest risk factor. The overabundance of food and possessions causes the chronic civilization sicknesses of today. Overeating is a sign of our spiritual hunger. Overconsumption of material goods becomes the ruin of society, and its values are upset and sometimes even destroyed. Hildegard sees horrible epidemic diseases for people who get stuck in materialism:

> I saw an enormous fire with gigantic black clouds and countless worms [infectious diseases]. Many people suffered here because they were occupied during their lifetime with financial and material wealth. They were blown from one place to the other by storms and winds. They burned in the smoky fire because they had lost the loving God, as they were so busy with themselves. Many of them were turned to stone by greed. Heavy blows and fire took all their fortune until they learned their lesson. (LVM)

People with too many worries lose their immune power and risk the possibility of autoaggressive sickness, which can come in many forms.

Spiritual Healing

Spiritual healing of fear, worry, and concern for the future resulting from the material concern for worldly things and leading to failure and frustration can be healed through fasting and physical exercise.

Follow the way to spiritual energy and freedom from worry by reading and praying Psalm 42, Psalm 55, Matthew 6:25–34, 10:19–20 and 1 Peter 5:7.

28. *Obstinatio*	*Compunctio cordis*
Obstinacy	**Remorse**
Hard-heartedness	Repentance
Pig-headedness	Regret
Stubbornness	Penitence, shame
Rigidity	Flexibility
Arrhythmia	Normal heartbeat
Caught in a rut	Ready for a new start

Crystal Therapy

The jasper is the heart stone to treat arrhythmia, irregular heartbeat, and heart pain.

Place the jasper on your heart until it becomes hot; remove it and let it cool down. Repeat as often as necessary. The jasper will remove excess energy from the heart in a few minutes.

Our heart is the center of our soul; it beats according to our emotions, our thoughts, and our actions. It beats faster in times of joy or rage than in times of rest, prayer, and meditation. During physical fitness it can beat 130 to 180 times a minute but also decrease to 40 to 50 times at rest, especially in athletes. You can bring your heartbeat down if you put your finger on your pulse and breathe very slowly and deeply. The rapid beating of the heart—in Latin *compunctio cordis*—is not a sickness, but rather a healing remedy that tells us, Wake up, you are in danger, turn around, start all over again.

Galangal and Jasper

You see how important it is to listen to your heart. Hildegard has two wonderful remedies to help you immediately out of a life-threatening situation, but they cannot change your life. A strong heart-pain reliever is galangal, a very hot spice in the ginger family. It is even more reliable than nitroglycerine. Leave it on the tongue until it disintegrates. The heart pain vanishes within 5 minutes, and this can prevent a heart attack. The herb is safe and has no side effects. You can repeat the procedure, leaving it on your tongue each time until the pain is completely gone. You might have to see a doctor or go into a hospital, but you have a much better chance of surviving than without the galangal.

Jasper is a precious stone that can be shaped into a handy disk 2 to 3 inches (6 cm) in diameter with a thickness of 1/8 inch (0.5 cm). The disk is cold, and when you place it on your heart when you suffer from arrhythmia, it takes away the excess energy and becomes quite hot. Put aside the disk until it is cool, then repeat 2 or 3 times until the heartbeat is normal again.

The heart is the center of the soul; it beats according to our emotions, our thoughts, and our actions. It beats faster in times of joy or rage than in times of rest, prayer, and meditation. During physical fitness it can beat 130 to 180 times a minute but also decrease to 40 to 50 times at rest, especially in athletes. You can bring your heartbeat down if you put your finger on your pulse and breathe very slowly and deeply. The rapid beating of the heart—in Latin *compunctio cordis*—is not a sickness, but rather a healing remedy that tells us, Wake up, you are in danger, turn aroud, start all over again.

People who misunderstand the beating of the heart go repeatedly to the doctor until she loses patience. Finally the doctor prescribes a beta-blocker, which cuts off the emotional feeling from the heart so that the heart is disconnected. Now these people can get excited without feeling the heartbeat, and many run around like this. The actor on a beta-blocker, for instance, has no stage fright, but his emotional energy is gone. As soon as we take the beta-blocker, we are chronic heart patients endangered by all the side effects.

No, the rapid heartbeat is no sickness; it is a remedy in times of peril and provides us with the power to change. It is the force we need for a new beginning if something goes wrong in our lives. If we overlook the heartbeat or don't even care, we run into trouble and anxiety and become hard-hearted. This can cause hardening of the arteries and lead eventually to a heart attack or stroke, the number-one killers today.

The immobile bull is a good symbol for obstinacy, which is a result of worry and anxiety about earthly matters. The stubborn bull can be very dangerous and kill you if you don't wake up and make a new start.

"Those who petrify internally are like death itself, which neither hears nor sees," writes Hildegard. "They cannot be awakened through the breath of God. Obstinacy is malicious. She is like a mole underground who turns the good upside down and runs stubbornly according to its will."

Stubborn people feel and act as if God does not exist. They do not take the trouble to understand others. They do not feel any compassion but instead injure other people with words sharp like arrows.

Harmful Words of Obstinacy

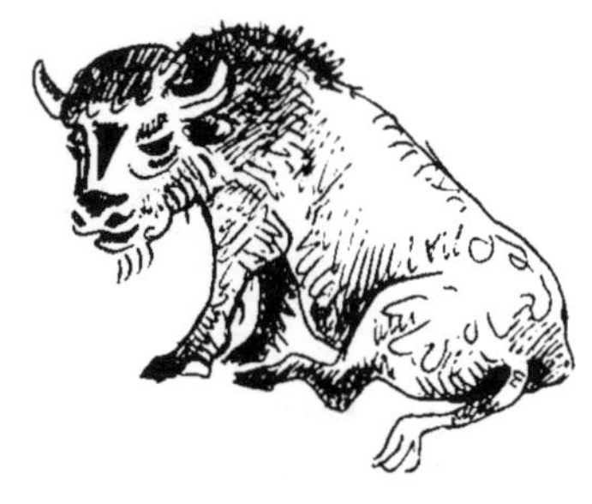

Obstinacy speaks bitter words:

"I don't care about unnecessary talk about various things and realities of life! When I speak, I do it with sharp, biting words. Nature also strikes the fruits and the ground with violent forces. I can profit only when I stay hard and inflexible. I don't care if I can't weep. To the contrary, let others drown in their own tears. Why should I work so hard? Why should I make any effort for something I can't attain? If someone strives for something that he can't attain, then it will be of no use to him." (LVM).

Changing our lives is not easy; sometimes it hurts to get out of our customary habits. We are faint-hearted and indecisive. We cannot let go of our problems; we carry our hurts and wounds throughout life because we cannot forgive. The wounds never heal and they make us hard until strong symptoms occur and we get very sick. If we can't let go and change, the sickness will return in many forms until we learn our lesson. Surgery and radiation can cut out the physical part, but the soul keeps burning. Many people take a tranquilizer, but chemistry cannot solve their spiritual problems. One day we must kill our bull of stubbornness so our wounds can finally heal forever. But we have to have courage and fight just like the prince who had to slash through the hedge of thorns before he could kiss the princess.

Healing Words of Remorse

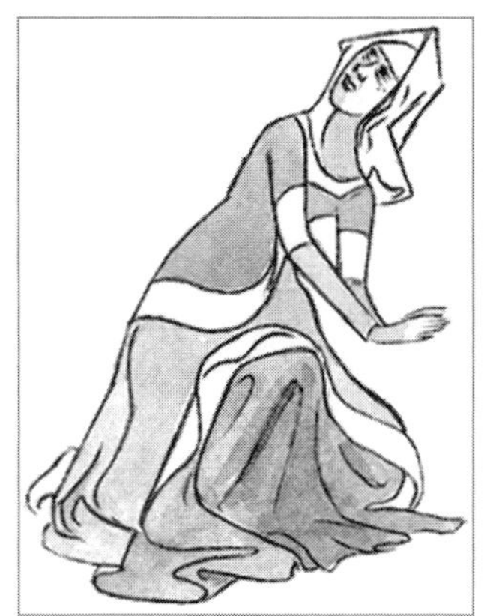

Remorse replies:

"You are entirely mistaken if you think you can succeed without effort. Look at the birds, the fishes, and the wild animals, see how they struggle for life. The young ones demand food from their parents just like the earth asks for life energy from the universe. God alone is the Father, because God is called on by all sons and daughters. They call on God because they get merciful help. When they ask for help, God gives freely. Why do you ignore me, God?

"I drink from God's radiant dew and on my knees I smile through my tears. Please help me, O God! I listen to the celestial harmony of the angelic spheres and shake off the clouds of hard-heartedness. Beyond the sunrise I receive God's radiant grace. And God endows me with spiritual nourishment and life energy because I ask for it. You, Obstinacy, receive nothing because you don't ask for anything" (LVM).

You can be entirely healed only if you look into the divine source whence healing energy comes. Look into the face of God as the eagle looks into the sun.

Organ Relationship

Obstinacy, hard-heartedness, stubbornness, callousness, pig-headedness, inflexibility, and arrhythmia relate to the pathology of the nervous system in the region of the sacrum, especially S4. The sacral nerve S4 controls the descending colon, the rectum, and the urogenital organs, especially the external genitalia, the prostate, the uterus, and the ovaries. (See Frank H. Netter, *Atlas of Human Anatomy,* plate 153, page 45.)

The same nerve controls the viscera and the iliac muscle, as well as the muscles of the hips, thighs, and legs; the lumbar plexus; the buttocks; and the arteries and veins of the legs and knees. This area is also responsible for the strength of the female and male sex organs.

In her vision of obstinacy, hard-heartedness, stubbornness, and inflexibility Hildegard sees fire and clouds full of stinging worms. The spiritual risk factors of obstinacy and stubbornness can give rise to inflammation and autoaggression of the organs, nerves, or muscles of this area.

> I saw an enormous darkness caused by burning tar and sulfur. Many people suffered in this place because they were obstinate, heartless, and stubborn during their lifetime. They burned in the dark fire because they lost their loving friendship with God. The were tortured with tar because they had lost their spiritual energy. (LVM)

People with too many worries lose the strength of their heart and suffer from diseases like arteriosclerosis, which can lead to angina pectoris or heart attack.

Meditation on Remorse

Remember the first day of Creation and its virtue *compunctio cordis.*

The first day of Creation has the power of revival and renewal and reminds us that each and every day is a new beginning. The cosmos carries the power of renewal through the angels. Hildegard writes that the light of creation contains an army of angelic spirits shining with great brightness. This spherical world of living angels *(viventes sphaeres sciliat angeli)* transports life energy from God to everything in the universe, on the earth, and under the earth to renew life and keep it alive. Angels are messengers, planetary spirits that help us fulfill our duties. The wings of the angels symbolize the intellectual power that emanates from God to humans. The angel of the first day brings light into the darkness so we can see clearly and return to God. This is the power of the new beginning and makes us cocreators with God for the new world to come.

Compunctio cordis, or the pounding of the heart, is incorporated in the body. It is not a sickness, but rather a remedy that carries the message: "Dear friend, return to God, return to love, you are at a dead end!"

Spiritual Healing

Spiritual healing for obstinacy, stubbornness, and heartlessness can be overcome by fasting and physical exercise. By falling on his knees, crying tears of atonement, and wearing a rough penitential robe, a fasting man has tools to transform obstinacy into true repentance of the heart.

Read and pray Jeremiah 15:19–21, sing the song of Psalm 98, and repent with the words of Psalm 109:21–31.

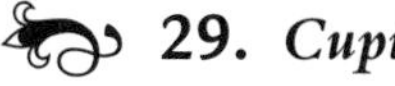

29. ***Cupiditas***	***Contemptus mundi***
Craving	**Letting go**
Desire for pleasures	Contempt for the visible world
Addiction	Liberation, freedom
Passion	Satisfaction
Obsession	Release
Imprisonment by one's habits	Independence
Enslavement	Rescue and redemption

Crystal Therapy

The sardonyx is used in crystal therapy.

Worn as a ring, sardonyx encourages freedom from obsession and addiction.

Americans believe they are endowed by their Creator with certain unalienable rights, among them life, liberty, and the pursuit of happiness, to live free and in harmony with themselves, with others, and with the entire universe. This is exactly the spirit of the liberation force, which can open our daily enjoyable prison of addiction and free us from obsessions in the visible world.

Always keep your eyes wide open for the treasure of the divine world, which is the core of your power center. The knowledge that we are a union of divine and human nature saves us from spending our life incarcerated in the jailhouse of the world.

Salvation is the key. Although *salvation* is one of those words that have lost their meaning for many of us, its roots go back to the Latin word *salvare* (healing, health, wholeness). Whatever metaphor we use to describe this feeling, we are in general agreement that this celestial power means "at-one-ment" of our souls with God. As soon as we forget the giver of life and freedom, we lose the energy and turn to the outside world to fill the gap.

Many of us spend our time and energy in filling the hunger of the soul with food from the world. Our souls become stuffed with material objects—money and an abundance of luxuries—which cannot be digested, and make us constipated and sick. All of this creates unhappiness and depression. The worst-case scenario begins when we try to overcome this misery with daily enjoyable poisons such as coffee, tobacco, sugar, alcohol, prescription drugs, and cocaine. Others try to fill the hole in the soul with work, books, computers, or sex. We put ourselves in our own prison, and some people can never escape.

Hildegard sees Craving as a sister of Obstinacy and Disharmony. People who live in a disharmonious and heartless environment escape to the prison of obsession.

Craving looks like a woman in a dark cloud; therefore, her feet are almost invisible. Her rapacity pulls her deep under the ground. She runs around like a hungry wolf, snapping everywhere for food. Her desire for goods increases her avarice to the point where she envies even herself. Her head is veiled in order to hide all her thoughts and intentions. She allows nobody to look into her heart. And she does not know the Golden Mean to bring back earthly and divine forces into harmony. Her desire to steal all kinds of treasures of the world is as big as the instinct of beasts and birds of prey. She is covetous, especially of the property of others. She commits malicious robbery for material as well as intellectual ownership. Her gluttony has no end. Nobody can help her, because she loves her dirty obsessions. She is so occupied with herself that she doesn't see God anymore but instead keeps her eyes on the business of others.

Harmful Words of Craving

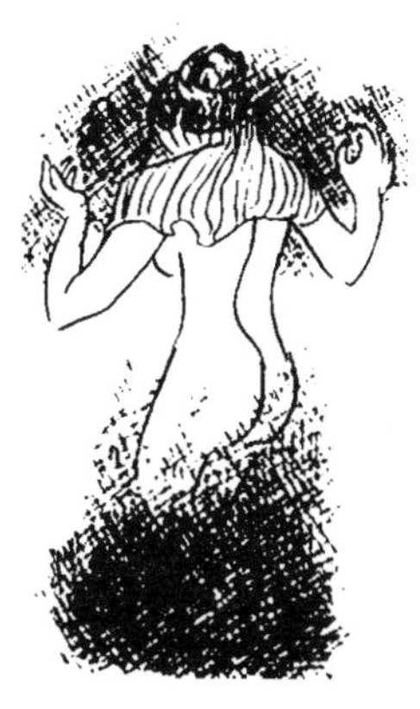

Craving is a grabby vice; it speaks:

"I have a great desire and an enormous drive to seize everything that is valuable, respectable, and beautiful. My prestige increases with every gift and possession, be it ever so small. The accumulation of possessions also increases my knowledge. With beautiful rings and splendid bracelets, as well as with other treasures, I am considered an upright, clever woman. Getting rich brings me security and stability. This way I have the feeling that I'm useful" (LVM).

Being rich is not security! Security comes from the appreciation of inner values, which are already there. Liberation is the relief from our addictions and obsessions, some of the major causes of unhappiness and disease.

The Spirit of God Opens the Dungeon of Addiction

We need extremely strong weapons to break through the prison of addiction and obsession. Hildegard describes a very dynamic power center, which is the foundation of our souls: the power of God's own Spirit. The term has nothing to do with the Holy Ghost, which can cause misguided people to think of a Halloween spook rather than God the Spirit helping us in our weakness.

The spirit is the giver of life that rippled over the face of water to create new human life as well as the universe. The same spirit can come swiftly to rock the boat like a hurricane or in kindness to open doors and prisons. In the same way, fire can be something terrifying or something warm and cozy, like the heat from a fireplace. Fire can also burn old habits and prisons. Whatever we call the spirit, it brings freedom and liberation to all of us—Buddhists, Hindus, Muslims, Jews, atheists—one and all.

Obsession and addiction are the most horrible bonds for all humans because they use the body and its desires to conspire against the soul.

Values from the visible world serve only the ego and cause us to question our very existence.

Many people fall into addiction through their insatiable desire to increase their prestige with wealth and possessions. They do this by questioning the sun, the moon, and the stars. They admire their astrologers as wise men. But how does this help? Where are all their possessions and property? Their things are in the abyss of hell, where they sit far away from the spirit of God and suffer the consequences of materialism. They have replaced God's spirit with matter; they rejected the divine and preferred throw-away goods.

Healing Words of Letting Go

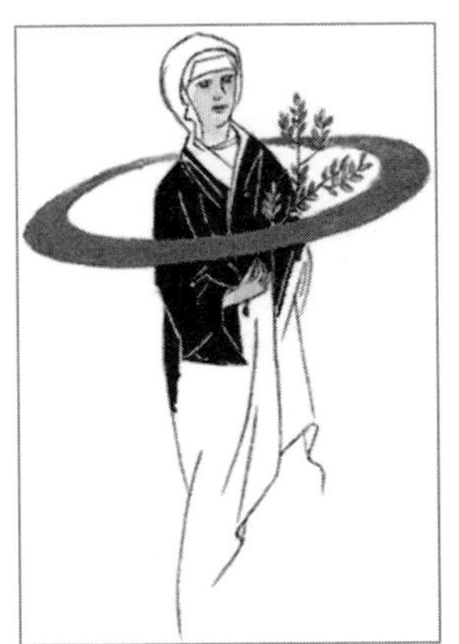

"You are weak and have no power to free me from misery. All suffering disappears through the fiery flames of the spirit of God and liberates me from all addiction. This lifts me and I fly up higher into another universe."

Letting Go continues:

"But I, Letting Go, make a conscious decision to seek the contact to the spirit of God who lives within. I follow my path with God and worship God as my Father. The burning fire of God's spirit is a purging fire for me in times of sudden attacks of addiction. I open my eyes to the fire of the spirit, who awakens me and moves me from prison to freedom. Even when people admire me as "the prince of the world" and give me all their treasures and resources to build my own paradise, I refuse. I need only my daily necessities. Everything else separates me from God. I blush when greediness returns" (LVM).

This "homecoming" to God is a transition from the temporal world to the divine.

The majority of people in the Western world get stuck with some addiction during their lives: drugs, alcohol, sex, work, cars, money, food—anything in excess. We live by fashionable manipulation and commercial propaganda. The most important message to us from Hildegard is to free ourselves from the pressure of addiction. Freedom from addiction and love for spirituality will heal neurosis and obsession. Modern cultural decay and civilization sicknesses are visible manifestations of an excess of material abundance and a hunger for love and spirituality.

Security often collapses as soon as our possessions are lost. True abundance comes not from amassing gifts or material things but rather from the celestial values that sustain life.

Here speaks Contempt, who opens our eyes to the gift of heavenly wisdom:

> I breathe life from the Giver of life. To convert greed into its virtue, man must begin to despise the world, holding it in contempt, scorning it, and defying it all the way to death itself.

"I will see to it that the conquering one eats from the tree of life which is in the paradise of my God. I will do so because the fountain of salvation, drowning death, poured its rivers upon me and made me green—fresh with redemption" (SC III, vision 10:13).

Organ Relationship

Craving, desire, addiction, and obsession are related to the pathology of the nervous system in the region of the sacrum, especially S5. The sacral nerve S5 controls the descending colon, the rectum, and the urogenital organs, especially the external genitalia, prostate, uterus, and ovaries. (See Frank H. Netter, *Atlas of Human Anatomy,* plate 153, page 45.)

The same nerve also controls the viscera and the iliac muscle as well as the muscles of the hips, thighs, and legs; the lumbar plexus; the buttocks; and the arteries and veins of the legs and knees. This area is also responsible for the stimulation of the female and male sex organs.

In her vision of desire, addiction, and obsession Hildegard sees boiling water, dragons, and evil spirits burning in fire. Spiritual risk factors like addiction and obsession can give rise to inflammation, infection, or autoaggression of the organs, nerves, muscles, and joints in this area.

> I saw an enormous boiling great sea of an extraordinary length, depth, and width containing horrible dragons and evil spirits. The unsatisfied obsessions burned in the people like embers and hurt like biting dragons. (LVM)

Meditation on Freedom from Addiction

A key metaphor for the work of Jesus Christ is the gift of salvation and liberation from the evil of addiction and obsession. When anything like eating and drinking is misused to relieve emptiness, it becomes an obsession. The master of the universe holds in his hands the sun, moon, and stars; the four elements; the twelve animals in four directions as spirit keepers; and all human beings. Man and woman are "a mirror of all God's miracles."

Hildegard's symbol of the universe shows Jesus as a young man holding the globe. The color red signifies that he and the Godhead are the origin of divine love, which embraces all creation. And what has this love done for you and me and the whole world? Jesus brought the gift of salvation and freedom. He freed us from sin, from sickness, even from death. Jesus established a new relationship to bridge the gap between us and God, for us and for our salvation. Salvation has to do with the well-being of the whole person. The carpenter from Galilee healed all kinds of sicknesses. Thanks to the presence of Jesus, Galilee was almost completely free of disease. "Jesus went throughout Galilee, teaching in the synagogues, preaching the good news of the kingdom and healing every disease and sickness." This has moved people all over the world throughout history.

But what about obsession and addiction? Is not any kind of addiction sooner or later going to lead to death and destruction? Once the trigger is released, addiction runs out of control. Addiction shows our inner emptiness and is a replacement for God. People who live in disharmony or in boredom are desperately looking for some sort of release: sex, work, money, drugs—whatever name you give it. All of this is an expression of spiritual hunger. The Latin word for alcohol also means "spirits"—the same word for the highest religious encounter as for the most horrible toxin. Or, as Carl Gustav Jung, the great master from Lake Constance, wrote: "Spiritus contra spiritum."

Only when we are ready to find and release the cause that evoked the disease will health come. When worse comes to worst, in the dead end of our deepest despair, when we have nothing in our hands to grasp and are starting to sink, and we are ready to give up everything that has been sweet and attractive, then we can fall into the hands of God and God will fill us with everything we were looking for.

Only Jesus the liberator saves and frees us from addiction; a change in a borderline situation can occur only through a supreme power. Remember, only the Master of the Universe is able to free us from whatever binds us. He changed the prostitute Mary Magdalene into a saint and the thief and murderer who died with him on the cross became the first man in paradise: "Today, you shall be with me in paradise!" What Jesus has done for us and our freedom and salvation is useful even today for everyone all over the world, for those who struggle, yearn, and search for the walk with God.

Spiritual Healing

Spiritual healing of craving can be reached through fasting, meditation, and physical exercise. In addition, Hildegard recommends generous gifts to the poor and active social work to overcome the daily habits of addiction.

Change the object of your desire by meditating on Psalm 40, 42, 73:23–28 and 1 Corinthians 14:1.

30. ***Discordia***	***Concordia***
Discord	**Concord**
Quarreling	Understanding
Disharmony	Harmony
Disagreement	Agreement
Dissension, friction	Bond, covenant
Opposition	Alliance
Instigation	Peacemaking
Separation	Unity, tolerance
Controversy	Accordance, consideration

Crystal Therapy

The aquamarine is the peacemaker stone.

Always wear an aquamarine (beryl), and hold and contemplate it often, and you will not quarrel with others but will instead remain calm and peaceful.

Everybody loves harmony, a feeling of wellness, and good team spirit. Some people are charismatic and increase the vibrations with jewels and body language. Emperors and kings used crowns and splendid garments to show their power fields. Ceremonial places and churches were built at sites with great vortex energy in order to fortify the power of the message. The art of creating a good atmosphere is practiced today in homes and gardens according to the principles of feng shui. But harmony is a natural thing and disappears with too much technique. The harmonious field can break down; thus, instead of being lifted up, a person can feel his energy being sucked away by someone weak.

Concord is actually the result of a constant energy flow from the mysteries of God to humanity. As shown in Hildegard's illumination of the Trinity, we can see the unspeakable expressed in a tremendous vision showing that we all are the visible image of the invisible God. We see a sapphire blue person surrounded by a pleasant fire of reddish gold. At the same time, a bright silver light surrounds this golden fire. All three shining colors represent simultaneously the power of the visible Christ (blue), the golden power of the spirit of God (like an electromagnetic field), and the silver-circled splendor of God, the One and Only. Hildegard calls this divine power center *lucida materia* or "shining matter," which awakens and fills with life the wild matter *(turbulenta materia)* to create the full energy spectrum. This event is the secret of life, when body and soul come together.

The body cannot exist without the energizing food of the soul. The soul, on the other hand, receives a continuous stream of higher energy from its divine origin. Through our interconnection to the divine we are able to receive energy and information, which are responsible for our well-being, the status of our health, and the exact functioning of our genetic cellular regeneration. Each of our ten billion body cells is endowed with all the information of a master library about how to build and maintain a human being.

Today we know from Albert Einstein's equation that matter and energy are one and the same. Just as Hildegard envisioned 850 years ago, energy *(lucida materia)* is matter *(turbulenta materia)* in movement. In scientific terms: $E = mc^2$; energy is mass times the speed of light squared. Energy animates the physical body and creates the human energy spectrum, which we enjoy as harmony. The relationship between body and soul, between matter and energy, is the key to understanding the nature of the universe, the relationship between God and humanity, and the forces of creation that link us with God and all other creatures.

Sometimes our harmony becomes disturbed through emotional stress, overwork, and negative feelings, with the result that the entire energetic field breaks down into virtually a blackout. The breakdown of energy can lead to catastrophic illnesses, as we can see in a heart attack, a stroke, or the failure of the immune system as in cancer and other autoaggressive ailments. When disease occurs, we know the energy flow of cosmic power is blocked. If people move away from the divine power and use the energy for their own personal satisfaction, it becomes very uncomfortable, and harmony changes into disharmony.

DISCORD: THE SISTER OF CRAVING AND OBSESSION

People who, in their gluttony for wealth fail to achieve what they really desire, sow the seed of discord become aggressive, like a vicious dog that attacks people.

In music one can hear discord as dissonance, which disturbs the ear just as disagreements disturb the soul. Discord enters the stage with a leopard head and a scorpion body and begins to argue against the Creator and the divine plan. She looks for her own advantage to control the universe and Creation according to her own will.

Harmful Words of Discord

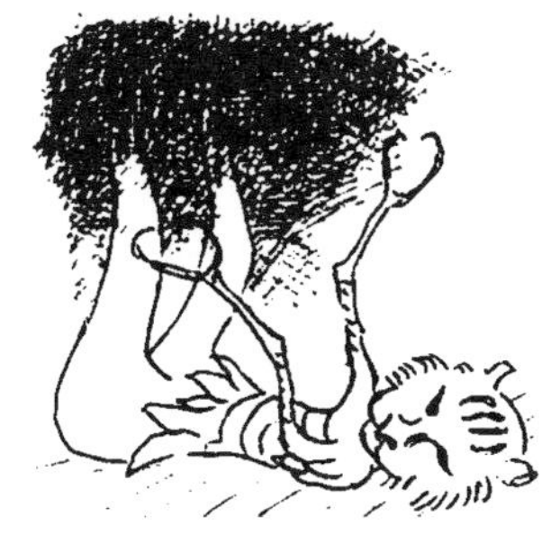

Discord speaks:

"I couldn't care less about the universe. The east keeps everything for itself; the south does the same. The morning sunrise glows golden, the west is darkness, and the north can darken the sunlight. I do the same! And what should I do with the animals, the birds, the fish, and the wild animals? I control their lives and use them for my satisfaction to obtain more power, to control other beings, and to accumulate more wealth. I live with all these creatures and decide what they are and how they can profit me. Noblemen and slaves, rich and poor, I turn all of them around like a wheel. Each will do what he wants and I do the same" (LVM).

Concord and harmony put discord in its proper place. It establishes balance and brings peace to all quarrels and feuds.

Healing Words of Concord

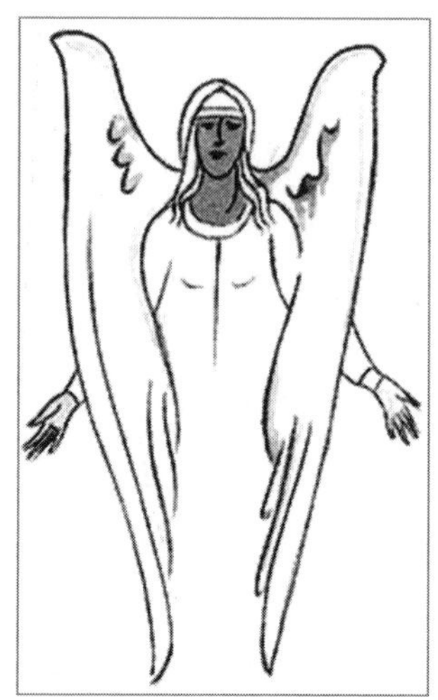

Concord responds:

"What person has so much strength that he or she tries to fight against God? And who has so much courage that he or she dares to plunder and destroy me with the ugliness of hate and envy? God alone is just and truly has power and glory. I want to embrace God always with a pure heart and with a joyful face. I always want to rejoice in God's justice. I do not, however, want to be changeable; I want to endure always with one soul and to praise God continuously. Therefore, neither the devil nor any evil person can soften me or hurl me down to foolishness or craftiness. Indeed, I will always persevere as an imitator of peace" (SC III, vision 10:4).

Organ Relationship

Discord, quarreling, disharmony, friction, and dissension are related to the pathology of the nervous system in the region of the sacrum, especially S5. The sacral nerve S5 controls the descending colon, the rectum, and the urogenital organs, especially the external genitalia, prostate, uterus, and ovaries. (See Frank H. Netter, *Atlas of Human Anatomy,* plate 153, page 45.)

The same nerve, S5, also controls the viscera and the iliac muscle, as well as the muscles of the hips, thighs, and legs; the lumbar plexus; the buttocks; and the arteries and veins of the legs and knees. This area is responsible for the strength of the female and male sex organs.

In her vision Hildegard recognizes the results for disharmony and discord in symbols related to fire, fog, horrible worms, and evil spirits.

> Quarreling people were pushed around from fire to darkness and back again, tortured by evil spirits. Horrible dragons bit these people, because they had lived in conflict with many other people. (LVM)

Spiritual Healing

Spiritual healing of discord and conflict occurs by fasting and exercising as well as by wearing a shirt made of coarse hemp. Extremely beneficial is the rejection of comfort and luxury.

Meditate on Psalm 133 and these Bible passages: John 17:22–23, Galatians 3:26 and 28, and Ephesians 4:2–6.

Chapter 7

The New Elders Ascend to the Summit

The positive outcome of our lives depends entirely on the art of changing the weakness and misery of old age into the beauty and strength of a wise man or woman. In order to become a spiritual elder, we continue our journey of learning using the last five powerful forces in our lives. The goal is the creation of a miraculous final unity of the purified opposites. Just as evening gives birth to morning, so out of darkness arises light, and by the same law of opposites conscious awareness of the negative creates the positive.

31.	*Scurrilitas* (scurrility, vulgarity)	*Reverentia* (Reverence)
32.	*Vagatio* (vagabondage)	*Stabilitas* (stability)
33.	*Maleficium* (occultism)	*Cultus Deus* (dedication to God)
34.	*Avaritia* (avarice)	*Sufficientia* (satisfaction)
35.	*Tristitia* (melancholy)	*Caeleste gaudium* (heavenly joy)

As we become older and realize the body is inevitably losing its health, our souls develop the greatest amount of spirituality and wisdom by remembering their life experiences. In contrast to today's practice when we treat aging as a terminal illness, the human soul can reach the highest summit of energy and joy. Hildegard herself was a remarkable example of the new "senior citizenship" due to her inspiring visionary and active work.

A Brief Biography

Life in the twelfth century was filled with suffering. Women left alone by their husbands, who went away to wars and the Crusades, faced poverty and hard work. Women's life span extended to only a few years after their child-bearing years. Upon raising their children, they had nothing to look forward to but preparing for death and the world to come.

Hildegard, however, lived an extremely long life. She died in her eighty-second year on September 17, 1179, honored by her contemporaries as a source of wisdom and spirituality. At the end of her life she told her last secretary, Wibert von Gembloux, "Whenever I'm occupied with my visionary work, I don't feel like an old woman but rather like a young girl." Her secretary added admiringly that she was completely transformed by her visionary gift.

When Rubertus, the abbot of Königstal, in Belgium, received Hildegard's letter he was so impressed that he exclaimed to friends, "I don't think I have ever heard such literary power and magnificence from any other teacher in France, not even those with intellectual greatness at the university in Paris."

Hildegard gained the energy for her remarkable activities from a breakthrough in consciousness emerging from her vision of earth and all of Creation. When she was sixty-five years old, she wrote her last cosmos-oriented theological book, *Liber Divinorum Operum.* In this book she describes humanity, in the center of the cosmic wheel, as God's most complete and beloved creation.

In her opening remarks she summarizes her cosmic spirituality. She viewed the presence of God as no less in nature than in spirit. The divine manifests itself in trees, water, clouds, wind, sunshine, and the whole universe. Hildegard saw our planet as a living and breathing organism with intelligence and radiance to sustain all life. We learn to live in great harmony with and respect for all of creation, enjoying the world and all fellow creatures in the here and now. She opens our eyes to the beauty and the presence of God in *this* world, because we are part of it and stand in the middle of the cosmic wheel.

With this creed Hildegard became the pathfinder of a new spiritual awareness as she created a global consciousness showing the interconnection of all men and women. She encourages us to have a more loving and respectful relationship with all life in the physical world. This gives us a foretaste of paradise.

Hildegard points out that although you cannot see the Creator, you can experience God in creation.

She writes: "I am the highest power, the fiery life power.

"I have ignited every spark of life, and I emit nothing that is dead. I fly above the earth with my lofty wings. I have put together the universe with wisdom. I am the fiery life of the divine essence. I flame beyond the beauty of the fields. I glitter over the water with radiance and burn in the sun, the moon, and the stars. I awaken everything to life with a breeze, as with invisible life.

"The air lives by turning green and blossoming. The waters flow as if they are alive. Full of life the sun shines, and after its disappearance the moon lives from the light of the sun. The stars, too, give a clear light, as if they were alive. I have established the pillars that bear the entire universe as well as the power of the wind and have selected lesser of weaker winds, which resist other mighty winds so that they do not become dangerous. In the same way the soul envelops the body and maintains it so that it does not die. And so I am hidden in every creature as fiery life. Everything burns from me like a wind-tossed flame in a fire. Everything lives from my essence and there is no death in it, for I am life" (LDO 1:1).

With this message Hildegard became a spiritual leader, a political adviser, and a teacher of the young. She attracted people like a magnet. Thousands came to seek personal counsel and she wrote more than three hundred letters to her contemporaries, including the emperor Frederick Barbarossa, many kings throughout Europe, eleven popes and numerous archbishops and bishops, as well as ordinary people. The cloister on the Rupertsberg became the meeting place of all Europe. Her convent attracted an increasing number of sisters, mainly from noble descent, whom she trained in the Benedictine way of life.

At the same time she founded a new convent on the other side of the Rhine River, in Eibingen, at Rüdesheim. Twice a week she crossed the Rhine in a rowboat in order to visit her new sisters. If we look at the flowing Rhine today, we are amazed at the strength of a woman who rowed the two miles across the river at the age of sixty-five.

In her concern for her mission, she traveled all over Germany, up and down the Rhine and along the Main and Mosel Rivers by boat, and on foot or by horse. In contrast to the beliefs of some modern historians, Hildegard was not fragile and ill with migraine headaches, but rather a well-trained, strong woman. Even at the age of seventy she traveled for days by horseback to the convent of Zwiefalten, close to Lake Constance, to speak in public.

Hildegard found the nation in spiritual despair. She fought against the politically corrupt church leaders and their materialism and sexual extravagances. The population suffered from terror and desperation. The pope and his army battled against the emperor Frederick I and his worldly authority.

A new spiritual movement of the Cathari emerged from these dark days in the Middle Ages, proclaiming that this world was the invention not of God but rather of the devil, with the pope his advocate. Hildegard confronted the Cathari: "It is not God who created the evil of the world. Evil is the result of failures of human beings not putting enough effort into changing the political life for the better."

We cannot destroy evil through war or burning heretics. Evil is there so that we search for the good. The hidden good behind all evil is the lesson to be learned and the purpose of our lives. She proclaimed very clearly: "Naturam homine bonum est!" (Mankind is good by nature!)

God has not made any mistakes. It is an insult to speak poorly of humanity and of Creation. This planet is home for all of us and we are all linked in the cosmic net. How wonderful this world is if we only give it a chance by working together now and enjoying the fruits of our lifetime here. Today we cannot live like Hildegard in her convent, but her visions can lay the foundation for a new stage of life, a bulwark throughout global changes and a powerful spirituality awakening. What a contrast to the useless elderly pushed away in old-age homes and set in front of a TV. Our seniors should become the spirit keepers for wisdom and spirituality. They must follow new ways in the future and be responsible for the safeguarding and survival of the spiritual life of the younger generation.

The Supreme Allroundman

Hildegard describes Jesus Christ turning around the universe to inspect all four corners, or directions. His feet are firmly established in the sea of the abyss, the base of life. This area is the workshop of God where everything on earth is prepared. The feet symbolize this region; they carry the body in a marvelous manner. Is there an architectural engineer on earth who could construct such a heavy mass as the human body balanced on two little feet?

The last five virtues and weaknesses are powers related to our feet. Hildegard describes the feet:

"They must attract everything, must clean everything, must hallow everything, must keep and carry everything, in order to penetrate everything in the world with the sweat of their dampness and strengthen all creatures in the same way, as the soul makes the body strong. . . . Man himself suppresses the force of the world elements found above the earth, on the earth, and under the earth with his feet" (LVM).

31. *Scurrilitas*	*Reverentia*
Scurrility	**Reverence**
Irreverence	Awe
Contempt	Appreciation, gratitude
Insult	Admiration
Shamelessness	Thankfulness
Obscenity	Dignity
Sarcasm, abuse	Esteem
Disrespect, debasement	High regard
Rudeness, disdain	Recognition
Arrogance, haughtiness	Modesty, gratefulness
Superiority, snobbishness	Simplicity, delight

Crystal Therapy

The gold topaz represents the presence of God, as gold is always the color of God.

Scurrility is characterized by the trickster, the practical joker or clown one meets everywhere. Like a crab with black hair he enters the scene ready to insult and abuse others with his tricks.

Harmful Words of Scurrility

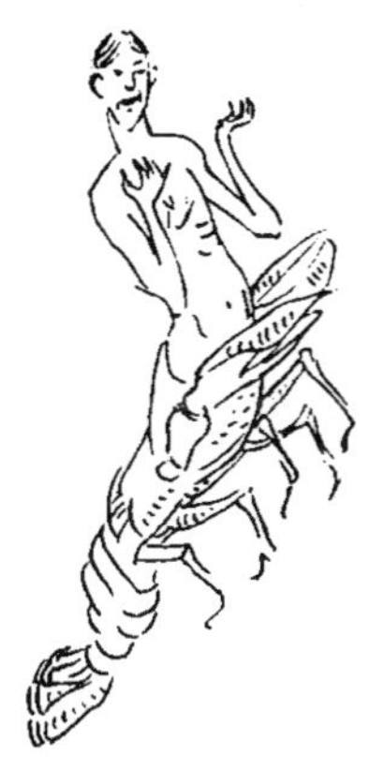

Scurrility speaks:

"Everyone has to live according to my rules. I am always there and decide everything according to my will. Most people are foolish and simple, to be neither regarded nor appreciated. I will catch them with my derogatory comments; the more I catch, the richer I will be. I will stretch my bow with the arrow of the big talker so that with only one word everyone will blush in front of me" (LVM).

The purpose of scurrility is to guide us to dignity and self-esteem. Nobody wants to live in an atmosphere of inferiority, unimportance, and worthlessness. The joy of life starts when we discover the golden, divine center, which is the core of our personalities. Through this golden sunshine in our souls we learn to appreciate ourselves and to recognize the value of others. This is exactly the message of reverence: Reverence is a feeling of profound awe, respect, and love. Reverence will accompany man from the high mountains of ecstasy and transformation to the deep valleys of worldly temptations and manipulation. Dignity and esteem for life protect us from looking down on creation and humanity and considering them as merchandise. We cannot see the human body as an object to buy or sell, raise embryos in test tubes, or sell babies or parts of human beings on the market.

Healing Words of Reverence

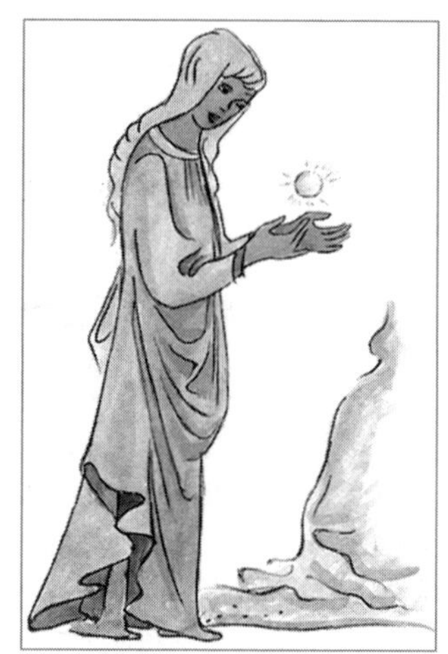

Reverence responds:

"Scurrility, you alarm everybody and fill people with anxiety and fear. If you only knew how life is created, you would not destroy it. You did not create life or give it its respect, dignity, and intelligence. In contrast to you, I am fascinated by the mountains and also enjoy a journey through the valleys and canyons. I walk among the highest and the deepest with joy and respect for creation. I don't hurt anybody, except you, you moron—I will stamp on you like dirt under my shoes. You earn nothing better, for you are the enemy of life: You neither admire nor esteem it; you hurt, damage, and ruin it" (LVM)!

As we grow older we ask ourselves, What is the purpose of life? What is its meaning? What is my contribution to this world? These are the final questions that many people today ask as the wise and the aged once asked in the past. We should remember the story of the rich young man who came to Jesus and asked, What is the purpose of life? Where is paradise? What makes my life meaningful? Real life starts, Jesus answered, when you do the most important thing in life: love the Lord your God with all your heart and with all your soul and with all your mind, and love your neighbor as yourself. Love yourself and mankind and the Creator of life—this is the message of reverence, dignity, and self-esteem as we go through life.

Organ Relationship

Scurrility and being rude, offensive, obscene, sarcastic, arrogant, cynical, and abusive, along with suffering from an inferiority complex—all relate to the pathology of the nervous system in the region of the coccyx, especially the coccygeal nerve Co2. This nerve controls the urogenital organs, especially the external genitalia, prostate, uterus, and ovaries, as well as the enervation of the feet and toes. This area is also responsible for the enervation of the female and the male sex organs. (See Frank H. Netter, *Atlas of Human Anatomy*, plate 153, page 45.)

In her vision of scurrility, shamelessness, irreverence, disrespect, disdain, contempt, and superiority, Hildegard sees the possible origin of inflammation and infections such as the autoimmune illnesses:

"I saw a raging fire with swarming worms. In the flames I saw the people who glorified offense and abuse and spoke outrageous, belittling, rude words of reproach during their lifetimes. They had to burn in the fire and suffer from worms because of their ignorance and obliviousness of God" (LVM).

People with a negative approach to life produce a lot of acidic black bile, which destroys the intestinal microorganisms, our first line of defense within the immune system. This causes leaky-gut syndrome—the migration of intestinal enemies into the bloodstream—and the production of too many immune weapons, which can destroy the entire body by autoaggression.

Spiritual Healing

Spiritual healing of scurrility and cynicism takes place by fasting, meditation, and stillness, which can change a negative lifestyles into the sunlight of reverence, dignity, and self-esteem. In this way we can detach ourselves from our selfish and life-denying lifestyles and enter loving, friendly, supporting relationships to enhance the quality of our aging.

Read Psalms 90 and 104 in a quiet corner prepared for the purpose of prayer, our own small temple or altar of peace. This will help us grow in reverence for all spirituality and human love. Our old age will be richer—our health will be strengthened, our memory improved, and immune weaknesses transformed into new energy.

32. *Vagatio*	*Stabilitas*
Vagabondage	**Stability**
Being labile	Being tough
Nervousness	Stamina
Anxiety	Tenacity
Restlessness	Steadfastness

Moodiness	Endurance
Being fickle	Being straightforward
Being aimless or purposeless	Having a goal
Being upset	Seeking balance of the spirit
Doubt	Perseverance

Crystal Therapy

The nature of jasper is stability, which reduces the negative humors affecting the intellect.

Place a piece of jasper in your mouth to improve concentration and sharpen your intellect. This therapy promotes steadfastness and stamina.

The vagabond is today's modern aimless person who is moody, labile, anxious, and upset in every respect. He changes his lifestyle as he does his clothing. The drifter looks in all directions to enhance life—different food, different clothes, and different habits, even in sex. Today he eats Chinese food, tomorrow Mexican. He wants to be treated with Ayurvedic medicine today, tomorrow with acupuncture, the next day with Hildegard's medicine. But he does not heal unless his spirit decides which way to go and stay. He is always dissatisfied and therefore on the move. He looks youthful, but is bald and has the face and beard of an old man.

Harmful Words of Vagabondage

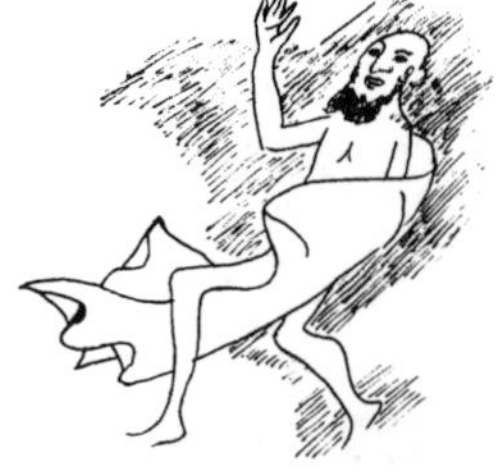

Vagabondage speaks:

"How stupid always to stay in one place with the same people. I want to be seen everywhere simultaneously so everybody can hear my voice [in the media]. My popularity and fame grow with my constant presence in public. Therefore, I like the way I am, with all my cleverness and smartness. In wisdom and intelligence I am like grass. I come into blossom and show myself here and there and everywhere in a complete self-presentation" (LVM).

Healing Words of Stability

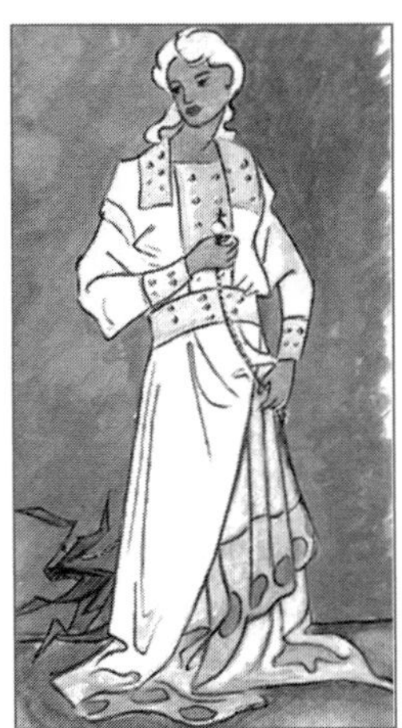

Stability protects us from being a labile nervous wreck:

"You, Vagabond, are a diabolic trickster! You will soon dry out with all your devilish attitudes as grass into hay. You will vanish like dirt on the road. In your inequity you are a voice of emptiness. You neither know the voice of wisdom nor speak the language of rationality. You jump back and forth like a grasshopper. You drift like a blizzard. You didn't try the food of wisdom, nor have you drunk wine in moderation. Your life is that of a homeless bird that never finds a place to land. You will never find rest because you will be burned to ashes and dust" (LVM).

Organ Relationship

The vagabond, or drifter—who is uneasy, neurotic, restless, moody, unstable, aimless, unpredictable, shaky, indecisive, and uncertain—is related to the pathology of the nervous system in the region of the coccyx, especially the coccygeal nerve Co3. This nerve controls sexual power, the urogenital organs (especially the external genitalia, prostate, uterus, and ovaries), and the enervation of the feet and the toes. (See Frank H. Netter, *Atlas of Human Anatomy,* plate 153, page 45.)

In her vision of the Vagabond, Hildegard recognizes that labile, nervous people possibly carry the origin of mental and intestinal disturbances. The chaotic change of the diet—today raw food, tomorrow fast food, the next day gourmet—causes a tremendous disorder in our intestinal microflora, with the result of indigestion, gas, heartburn, and either diarrhea or constipation. Our immune systems cannot heal if we try acupuncture first, then chemotherapy, and later Hildegard's medicine. The accumulation of contrasting belief systems from all over the world leads to mental garbage and spiritual trash. The more garbage we dump inside, the more we produce outside. If we don't look for our personal roots and grow, we decay.

I saw a great garbage pile heaped with rot and filthy dirt. Stinky gases emerged and spread all over. In this place I saw those people who were

> filled with instability and were restless throughout their lifetimes. They had to live in this swamp because of their great mistakes, burdened with guilt. They suffered from the smell because of the scourge of being a restless vagabond. (LVM)

Meditation on Stability through Love

Once we get in touch with our golden divine center, we learn to love ourselves and connect to the unlimited reservoir of God's love, which will overflow in us with joy. Hildegard chooses for this timeless, constant flow of love strong erotic symbols such as beauty, songs, kisses, and hugs in order to open all five senses. Each of us has a deep desire for love that creates a place of security, homeland, and stability. God has created every creature with this original love and faithfulness. The divine eternal love is based on commitment, like a mother's to her child, a dog's to its puppies, and a bird's to its nestlings.

Love without commitment produces instability and restlessness, and is all too common today. As soon as we transform our inner vagabond into a lover of God, we receive tremendous vitality and universal love, which can heal and strengthen the old body and also recycle negative energy into positive. Committed love can even transform an enemy into a friend through respect and honor. Committed love is holding what we love in esteem and reverence.

Spiritual Healing

Spiritual healing of Vagabondage takes place through fasting, physical fitness, and returning to God with the spirit of repentance. Garbage can be turned into compost! We can recycle negative energy into positive. We can transform the shaky lifestyle of the drifter into the power of stability, endurance, strength, courage, stamina, and trustworthiness.

As we practice spirituality and divine love, we will learn to overcome our physical debilities by opening our eyes to the beauty and love of God.

Reading Psalms 91 and 121 can be a big help in your transformation. We must learn to detach ourselves from our restless lifestyles and enter into more love and friendship during our elder years.

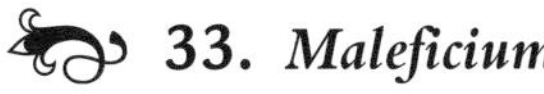

33. *Maleficium* **Occultism**	*Cultus Dei* **Dedication to God**
Psychotherapy without God	Divine spirituality
Magic, astrology	Reliance on God
Satanic cult	Devotion to God
Idolatry	Worship of God
Blasphemy	Adoration of God
Black magic	Devoutness for God
Scientism	Knowledge of God
Disregard for God	Cherishing God
Acculturation (loss of culture)	Culture, true religion

Crystal Therapy

The amethyst symbolizes the absence of all evil, which is portrayed by poisonous snakes.

Wear the amethyst as a ring or necklace.

If God is not the center of your interest, the center becomes vacant and loses its energy. This void screams for a replacement until the emptiness is filled. More and more people who have lost the divine orientation in their life are looking to psychotherapy as a replacement for religion and spirituality. The result is a new branch of an intellectual psychotherapy, which started in the last century with the psychoanalysis of Sigmund Freud and continued with the behaviorism of today's American educational system. The result is a pseudoscience from different schools of thought all contradicting one another. Not one school offers more healing results than does a simple placebo. Furthermore, in some cases people without psychotherapeutical treatment were mentally more stable than those with treatment. It is a fact that we cannot fill the divine center with man-made theories; it just does not work. The blackout continues and the hunger for a replacement becomes even stronger. The void is always there and can be filled only with inner values like God, love, trust, adoration, and commitment.

The third pair of vices and virtues divide mankind into the cult of God and the cult of the devil. Attached to the cult of the devil, with its sick-making practices, are such things as magic, sorcery, and witchcraft. Black is every witch, black her cat on the broomstick, black her magic. These lack the light of Christ's love. This vice has a wolf's head, a lion's tail, and a dog's body.

Harmful Words of Occultism

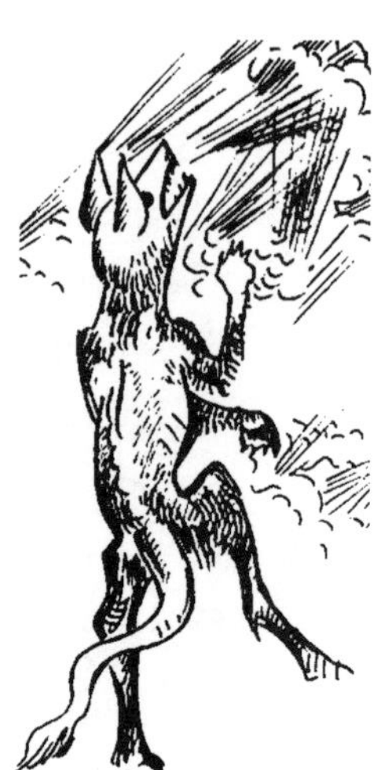

Occultism, who is playing with the Vagabond, speaks:

"I can talk a lot about Mercury and the other planets. I could even speak about all kinds of other things including philosophy. I have explored and discovered everything partly with the help of God, partly with my own research, and even through black magic. Who cares? For this reason I gave myself the names of the planets, received great wisdom, and made numerous discoveries about the sun, the moon, and the stars. But I, I manipulate and command the world and its people. I am the master of the universe. I rule over the stars of the universe and heavens, over the trees and herbs, over life and life energy. I command the wild animals and all the remaining living creatures on earth, as well as the worms above and under the earth. Who can stop me from my research? God has created everything. It is his will to explore and exploit the universe. It is stupid and senseless not to reveal all the secrets of life and make use out of them" (LVM).

Our scientific, high-tech world is full of magic. We believe in the latest scientific results and everything that is scientifically proved, even if it is to our own detriment. Try the magic pill, it keeps you happy and solves your problems—just ignore the side effects. We take beta-blockers that cause stroke, increase heart pain, and bring on a heart attack. We swallow painkillers that cause internal bleeding and ulcers, and we take chemotherapy that kills our immune systems. We use mobile phones that microwave our brain and eat an abundance of food that ruins our health. But even worse, we have lost our own strength and identities and have become a boring carbon copy of the mass of society. Our centers are empty and we look desperately for something to fill the void, like money, sex, new things, luxuries, and drugs.

Healing Words of Dedication to God

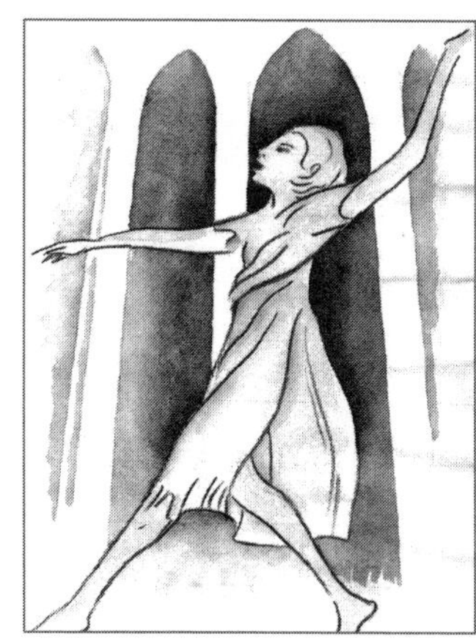

In reply to Occultism, Dedication to God answers:

"What is more pleasant to God, to honor him or his creatures? The creatures, originating from the Creator, cannot bring anything to life. And what is life, created by God? Man and woman have rationality; the rest of the world is made up of natural elements. Humanity exists and lives from its rationality, whereas all the others exist by their natural instincts. And so humanity has a certain tone to its intelligence, whereas all the others are silent. They can help neither themselves nor others.

"But you, Occultism, you are only a ring without a center. You performed many studies in nature, but creation itself refuses to respect you and will reclaim its possessions. You killed the name of God in yourself; therefore, you will be thrown into hell like a stone. All the people will accuse you because you guided them into blasphemy and profanity. You led them astray, hurt them, and took away their divine treasure" (LVM).

Organ Relationship

Occultism, magic, acculturation, idolatry, blasphemy, irrationality, and disregard for God relate to the pathology of the nervous system in the region of the coccyx, especially the coccygeal nerve Co4. This nerve controls sexual power; the urogenital organs, especially the external genitalia, prostate, uterus, and ovaries; and the enervation of the feet and the toes. (See Frank H. Netter, *Atlas of Human Anatomy,* plate 153, page 45.)

In her vision of magic and occultism, Hildegard sees the possible origin of mental and intestinal disturbances. Because we have lost the ability to worship our divine centers and therefore no longer have their energy, many diseases are now incurable.

> I saw a great swamp burning with a bubbling fire and a terrible odor where squirmed countless snakes and worms. Here I saw those people who mixed potions, did magic, and used diabolic wiles to trick their fellow men during their lifetime. They had to live in this swamp because they had lost their original faith in God. (LVM)

Meditation with the Gold Topaz

Evoking the Power of the Golden Divine Center (SC, vision 2:5)

Remember that the body is the visible house of the invisible God who lives deep within us. Our bodies are not our real personalities. When we go deeper into ourselves, we reach our souls, which are the golden divine center inherent in all humans. Here we discover the presence of the Trinity—the creative power of God, God's loving hope in Jesus Christ, and the enthusiasm and eagerness of the spirit—which provides us with infinite life energy. Together with the four elements they furnish all the life energy we need to survive.

When we remember these seven forces, strong energy flows throughout the entire body and healing occurs. We are at one with God and with the universe. We become aware of our uniqueness but also of our interconnectedness with the rest of humanity, all creatures, and the entire universe through the cosmic internet. Some of us have a hard time finding this divine center because we feel stuck in our bodies and have forgotten our souls and our original home in God. No one has ever seen the soul, but simply by looking in the eyes of others it is possible to get a glimpse.

Remember Hildegard's words:

> There are three powers in the stone, three in the flame, and three in the word. In the stone are moist greenness, tangibility, and a red fire. It has moist greenness so that it cannot be destroyed, tangibility for defense, and a reddish fire to give heat. The moist greenness signifies God, who never becomes dry. The tangibility stands for Jesus Christ, who was able to be touched and grasped. The red fire signifies the Spirit of God who is the guardian and illuminator of the hearts of faithful people. . . . As these three powers are in one stone, so is the true Trinity a true unity. (SC 2:2)

Discover Your Own Soul

You can create a ritual to help discover your soul.

- Find your favorite place at home or in nature.
- Remove or change your clothes in order to become a spiritual flying eagle.
- Light a candle.
- Sit still in a chair, lie quietly on the ground or floor, or stand silently for a period of time.
- Take deep breaths and relax.
- Let go of everything that disturbs you.
- Go deeply into yourself and connect with the seven forces of your soul.
- Rejoice and praise to evoke the divine power.

Spiritual Healing

Spiritual healing of occultism, magic, scientism, and psychotherapy without God is possible through fasting, physical fitness, and returning to God in the spirit of repentance.

The afflicted will find additional help by reading, praying, and meditating on Habakkuk 2:18–20 with its awe-inspiring last verse, "The Lord is in his holy temple: Let all the earth be silence before him." It is worthwhile to compare this Old Testament text with I Corinthians 3:16–17: "For the temple of God is holy, which temple ye are." Psalms 84, 99, and 100 awaken in us the yearning for our home in God and guide us to consecration, devotion, and true worship.

Gold Topaz Prayer

Press a golden topaz on your heart and say:

"God, who is above everything and magnified in everything, with great respect to you, do not push me away, but rather keep me, strengthen me and become one with me, in your blessing."

Or in Latin: "Deus, qui super omnia et in omnibus magnificatus est, in honore suo me non abjiciat, sed in benedictione me conservet, confirmet, et constituat."

Then praise and rejoice with Psalm 103:

Praise the Lord, O my soul;
all my inmost being, praise his holy name.
Praise the Lord, O my soul
And forget not all his benefits.
Who forgives all your sins and heals all your diseases,
who redeems your life from the pit,
and crowns you with love and compassion,
who satisfies your desires with good things,
so that your youth is renewed like the eagle's.

Words are very powerful, especially holy words. When you celebrate this power ritual, you receive access to unlimited energy. You feel magnificent, uplifted like an eagle. Your soul grows wings and you become a messenger between heaven and earth.

---

34. ***Avaritia***	***Sufficientia***
Avarice	**Satisfaction**
Selfishness	Benevolence
Insatiability	Abundance
Ravenousness, gluttony	Satiation
Miserliness	Generosity
Covetousness	Gratitude
Possessiveness	Detachment
Desire	Contentment
Craving	Letting go

Crystal Therapy

Due to its origin from fire, air, and water the agate increases sensitivity, gratitude, and the ability to let go.

Practical application has shown that an agate necklace worn at the time of the full moon calms the impulse and habit to drink, to steal, or to run away during that time.

When psychotherapy fails, as an act of desperation we try to fill the emptiness of our soul with wealth and possessions. Avarice is the driving force to harm and betray others to get more and more. No matter how much we have, if we are greedy, we want more and more private property.

Why is it that economic success does not necessarily bring personal contentment? asks *Time* magazine journalist Gerd Behrens in his essay "Healthy, Wealthy, and Unhappy." Wealth breeds unhappiness. The key question, "Are you happy?" shows that the poorest Europeans, the Irish and the Portuguese, are the most content, whereas the richest Germans were the most miserable. Wealth and happiness are contradictive because we cannot feed the hungry soul with objects from the outside.

Materialism does not fill the hole in our soul. The emptiness continues and the hunger for a replacement begins to take different forms—sex, cars, money, designer clothes, food, alcohol, and drugs, for example. Each desire creates a new one. As soon as we lose all our possessions, our health, or our status, we can see that the void was always there and can be filled only by values from our own inner development: selflessness, readiness to serve others, self-sufficiency, and an inner peace of mind. The negative energy of greed has the mandate to open the prison doors to a positive state of mind filled with modesty and satisfaction.

Avarice has no hair on his head and sports a goatee. Through his nose he aggressively breathes in and out. His legs are bloody; his feet are like lion paws. His garment is white interwoven with black threads. A black vulture has its claws hooked into his chest. He leans against is a tree with its roots in hell, and its fruits are apples made of tar and sulfur, which this character devours greedily. All around him numerous horrible worms are crawling.

Harmful Words of Avarice

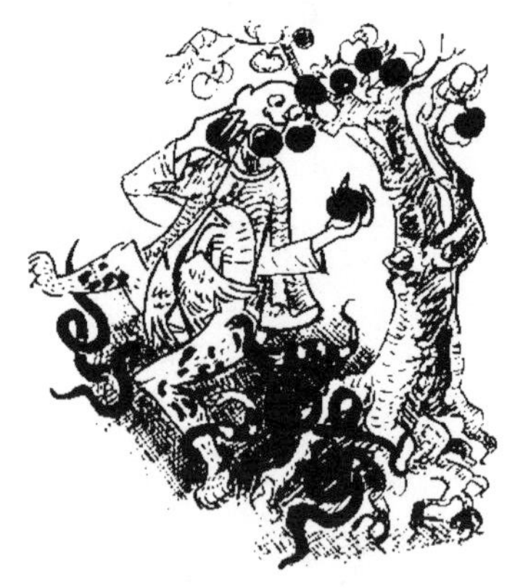

Avarice speaks in a mean voice:

"I am not a fool! At least I am smarter than those who wait for the wind and expect their livelihood from the air. I grab everything and gather it in my lap. There is nothing wrong in taking away the riches from a person who already has more that he needs. When I have as much as I want, worries will no longer plague me. Then I will not have to fear anyone, but rather will live off the fat of the land and have no need to beg my fellow man for sympathy. I am not a thief and a burglar. I take with the help of my talents only those things that I deserve" (LVM).

Avarice profits when people fight against each other and he can create increased sorrow and worry. People who are enslaved to greed have no security and stability because they are not rooted in God.

Satisfaction continues:

"You fool! This very night your life will be demanded from you. Then who will get what you have prepared for yourself? This is how it will be with anyone who stores up things for himself but is not rich in the things of God."

We are the mirror of God. He loves us with erotic love, with kisses and hugs like a lover adores his beloved.

Healing Words of Satisfaction

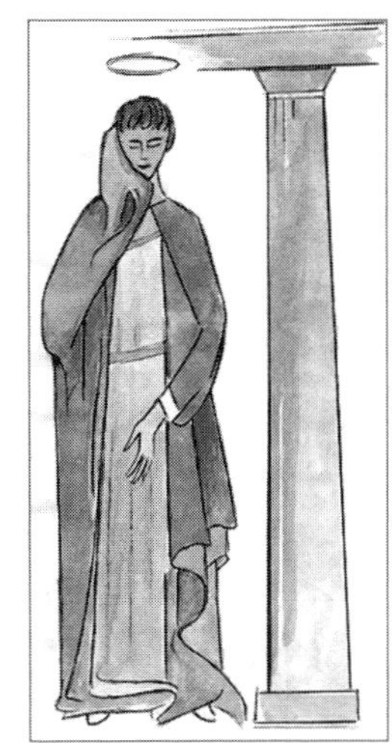

Satisfaction knows that the real inner treasure is our divine nature:

"O you devilish snare! Like a wolf you watch for prey; the property of others you devour like a vulture. Your huge boils like the humps of a camel burst open with pus as you are loaded with your forbidden desires. You are like the open throat of a wolf that swallows everything. You fell into the death valley of your unmerciful hard-heartedness and were deserted by God. Your behavior is cruel and heartless; you don't care about your fellow citizens. You live a miserable life and hide like a worm under the earth, as you reject heavenly values.

"But I, I soar above the stars and take pleasure from the divine gifts. I enjoy the music of the kettledrums, for I trust in God. I kiss sunshine when I embrace my God. I enclose the moon in my heart when I hug my God with affection. I am content with all that grows through the sun and moon. I am satisfied and have enough to exist. I live with everybody in compassion. Because I have mercy for everything, my robe is of white silk decorated with precious jewels. I live in the palace of the king and lack nothing my heart desires. I will partake of the king's banquet, for I am the king's daughter.

"But you, you unworthy fellow, you can run all around the earth and you still will never be satisfied. Take care who you are" (LVM)!

Where are the tyrants who oppressed and enslaved the people? They are all dead and decaying in the desert. They lived oblivious to the beautiful symphony and harmony of the spirit of God. They lost their joy for the divine and invisible and desired only material goods and visible objects. They did not care about salvation and the needs of their soul, which is why they are dead as charcoal, and why all their greedy works will die with them. Impulsive forces lead people into these lustful passions and teach them to grab as much as they can.

Organ Relationship

Avarice, miserliness, selfishness, insatiability, desire, possessiveness, craving, and attachment relate to the pathology of the nervous system in the region of the coccyx, especially the coccygeal nerve Co3. This nerve controls sexual energy; the urogenital organs, especially the external genitalia, prostate, uterus, and ovaries; and the enervation of the feet and the toes. (See Frank H. Netter, *Atlas of Human Anatomy,* plate 153, page 45.)

In her vision of the miser, Hildegard sees people with destroyed intestinal microflora, which causes weakening of the immune system. The resulting infections of various organs are described in visionary metaphors like burning fire related to fever and cruel worms as symbols for bacteria and viruses.

> I saw a fiery area that burned and glowed like hell. Numerous bloodthirsty worms were being blown about by the wind. Those people who accumulated foreign goods during their lifetime had to suffer in the fiery storm cloud. They had to burn in this fire because of their greed. The miser, who had damaged and injured his fellow citizens, was being attacked by the aggressive worms. (LVM)

People who steal the property of others suffer extreme fever attacks. The deep black hole in the ground symbolizes manic-depressive seizures.

> I saw a very deep well with a turbulent flame moving in and out of the fountain. It was so deep that I could not see the ground. Robbers, who had trespassed against others, burned in the flames screaming: "Why were we so cruel?" They were thrown in and out of the burning fountain because of their brutality. (LVM)

In her vision of theft Hildegard sees unexpected events like accidents, mental breakdowns, psychotic attacks, and epileptic fits.

> I saw a large and deep hole in the ground filled with many restless demons. They had to suffer because they had stolen during their lifetime. They could not leave the deep cavity and were attacked by numerous worms because of their nightly thefts. They were also attacked by demons because of their blindness toward God. (LVM)

Spiritual Healing

We can transform the greedy lifestyle of Avarice into peace of mind and satisfaction. Even thieves have a chance to be transformed if they give up their brutal lifestyle. As we practice the spirituality of letting go and being content, we can change craving and possessiveness into divine love, because God loves the remorseful lawbreaker.

According to the balance of cosmic law, everything we do—good or evil—comes back to us as good or evil. There is justice in creation and God is mild in his judgment. He joyfully welcomes the penitent wrongdoer (in the parable of the lost son, for example), but he punishes the sinner who cannot and does not repent. Nothing evil and unjust proceeds from God. He fights against everything bad, suffering like a fish on a hook, and not wanting to harvest what he didn't sow. He even goes into hell and takes out the sinner, if he so desires, because he likes to trick the devil. He also likes to help the nonbeliever be converted and filled with awe and praise. This he promised to all those who wanted to be saved and cleaned from greediness (LVM).

Fasting is the universal remedy to transform avarice and lust into satisfaction and contentment. During fasting we give up the habit of eating three times a day and learn to achieve happiness and obtain more energy without food. In contrast to fasting, eating creates a constant state of discontent; we eat and want more and more without being satisfied.

Fasting in combination with strong physical exercise teaches us to open our hands wide and let go of greed. Simultaneously during fasting we learn forgiveness and how to reconcile with those who have trespassed against us. We want to remember that God is willing to give us everything we really need.

In the same way, the negative energy of theft can be converted into the positive energy of good-heartedness during fasting. As a constant reminder, one should wear a scratchy hemp shirt.

"Theft out of greed can be changed into generosity during fasting, physical exercise, and praying for forgiveness on the knees" (LVM). *Reading and praying Psalm 90, especially verse 14, and Psalm 103, especially verse 5, are additional aids. And it is wise to learn by heart Philippians 4:11–13 and Hebrews 13:5.*

35. *Tristitia*	*Caeleste gaudium*
Melancholy	**Heavenly joy**
Sadness	Gladness
Misery	Rapture
Fear, anguish	Bliss, elation
Dejection	Blessing
Depression	Heavenly well-being
Gloom	Exultation
Pain and suffering	Triumph, ecstatic joy
Distress, agony	Rejoicing
Melancholy	Celebration
Grief	Jubilance
Black bile, blues	Festivity

Crystal Therapy

The onyx and the amethyst are strong stones against melancholy.

When you feel sad or depressed, look at an onyx and hold it in your mouth—all sadness will depart. Or wear an amethyst set in a ring or necklace, because negative thoughts and feelings flee this stone.

Weltschmerz (meaning "world pain" or "world-weariness"), sadness, and depression are all painfully familiar words to people afflicted with melancholy. Melancholy and Weltschmerz are the enemies of joy and happiness. However, we must consider the degree to which we experience these emotions. All of us feel down on occasion, when we have failed a task, have not achieved a goal, or are struck by a loss. Sometimes we feel like we're on top of the world but at other times we feel as if we're going through hell on earth. There is certainly no such thing as constant equilibrium of mood or of happiness.

Hildegard is concerned with the men and women who have forgotten the joy of heaven and instead attempt desperately to find happiness within their own harsh world. It is not surprising that they are overcome with apathy and hopelessness when confronted with the pain and suffering of the world. Hence, they fall prey to depression and lose all sense of hope. This pessimism results in the loss of divine joy.

Melancholy and depression can escalate to such an extreme that they lead to utter desperation and, in the worst case, even death. This is why depression cannot be cured by antidepressants. To the contrary, sometimes these medications give the patient just enough energy to actually end his or her own life. Healing powers always come from heaven and have their source in a rapturous divine joy, supported by Hildegard's visionary medicine, which neutralizes black bile, the cause of this affliction.

ABOUT GRUESOME MELANCHOLY

The worst of all vices culminates in melancholy. Humankind forgets its memories of God and loses its heavenly home. Neither the people themselves nor their friends, nor nature can instill a sense of joy anymore. This deficiency causes disease. Grief does not find pleasure in its divine home; it sees no value in the blooming power of life. Everything it touches is destroyed. Therefore, it laments: "I know of nothing at all with its home in God."

And so all vitality dies in the depressed, because the spirit of life has vanished. The afflicted person constantly attracts more sadness and in his despair neither speaks to his friends nor reconciles with his enemies. He internalizes all the pain of the world and hides behind his own difficulties, dodging all challenges and confrontations. He is like the dead in not looking up to his heavenly home and not trusting life itself.

God answers him: "I have created the sun, the moon, and all creation, and I have made human beings rational creatures. Therefore, you should recognize and love me freely from the bottom of your heart. You should not mistrust me and fight against me. Good is much better for you than evil. If you do not want to know anything about me, you cannot receive the gift of complete happiness. I have shown humankind its sanctity and its home. But all have ignored and abandoned me with their mistrust. And so in my desire to punish I must scrutinize and examine them and pass judgment in a righteous trial, because they were derogatory and have not accepted the good I have shown them."

VISUAL REPRESENTATION OF MELANCHOLY

Hildegard envisions Melancholy as a man in the figure of a woman who has regressed into a caricature. In his futility he embraces dry branches and curses the days of his life: "If only I had never been born."

This figure is entwined in the shriveled branches of a tree, just as this vice is surrounded by the contradictions it causes. One branch is covering his head, showing that remorse, which is the new beginning and the summit of all human understanding, is suppressed. Another branch winds around the neck and throat and portrays the fear that destroys all strength and energy with which he could endure suffering of the heart and be able to search for the bread of life. Yet another branch of the tree encircles his left arm, so he cannot move his arms but instead draws them to his chest, showing the fear and apprehension he has about eternal and spiritual works.

His hands jut out from the tree with nails like the claws of a wild animal, because all of his doings within this prison are disdainful and arrogant, and in a crude and savage manner they act with sinister greed and ruthlessness. The branches also signify an intense fear of death filled with horror, so these individuals lose the ability to work and live in peace. As a consequence, they lack the serenity necessary for studying and learning and use their free time instead to cultivate the sadness of their hearts. Depressed people are incapable of loving themselves or others; they have no belief in themselves and no self-esteem on either happy or sad days.

There are branches to both sides of the figure covering his stomach, because everywhere he surrenders to his world pain there appears doubt, despite the fact that he could guard himself against melancholy by virtue of his own intelligence. In situations in which he should effortlessly fend off carnal desires, the weakness of his soul causes him to plummet back into deep sadness once again. Neither God nor the world can infuse in him any sense of delight anymore.

Harmful Words of Melancholy

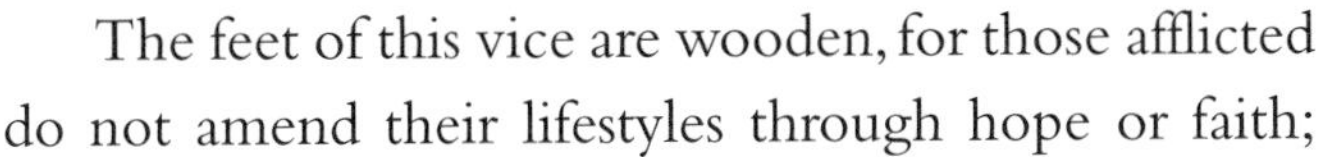

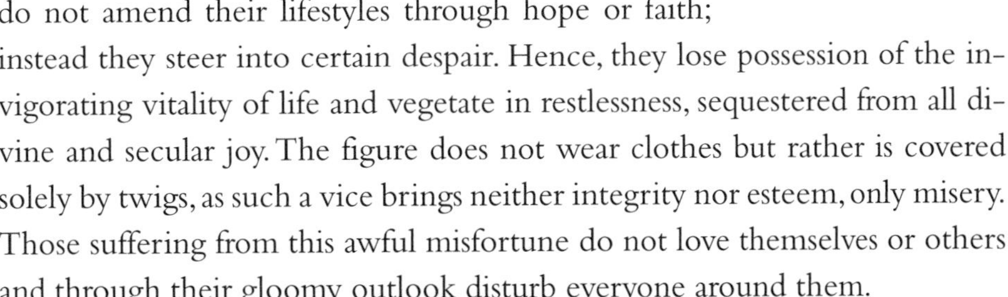

Melancholy speaks:

"Oh, had I never been born! What a life! Who will help me? Who will delight me? If God knew me, surely he would not bestow on me such misery. I have never received anything good that would cause me to trust in God" (LVM).

The feet of this vice are wooden, for those afflicted do not amend their lifestyles through hope or faith; instead they steer into certain despair. Hence, they lose possession of the invigorating vitality of life and vegetate in restlessness, sequestered from all divine and secular joy. The figure does not wear clothes but rather is covered solely by twigs, as such a vice brings neither integrity nor esteem, only misery. Those suffering from this awful misfortune do not love themselves or others and through their gloomy outlook disturb everyone around them.

From out of a dark cloud appear evil spirits with a dreadful stench. They pull those afflicted out of any potential consolation and equilibrium of mood. And so they curse themselves out of sheer desperation and hopelessness, robbing themselves of any belief in well-being.

More Harmful Words of Melancholy

Sighing, the figure leans back and speaks again:

"Even though I do rejoice in God, this gruesome feeling will not vanish. I have often listened to philosophers who praise the goodness of God. All in all God has not provided me with anything good. If God feels for me, why does he conceal his mercy from me? I would trust and believe in him if he would bequeath me something good. I don't even know who I am. I was born into calamity and created for sadness, living, as I do, without consolation. Oh, what good is life without friends and why was I born, when nothing good ever befalls me" (LVM)?

Healing Words of Heavenly Joy

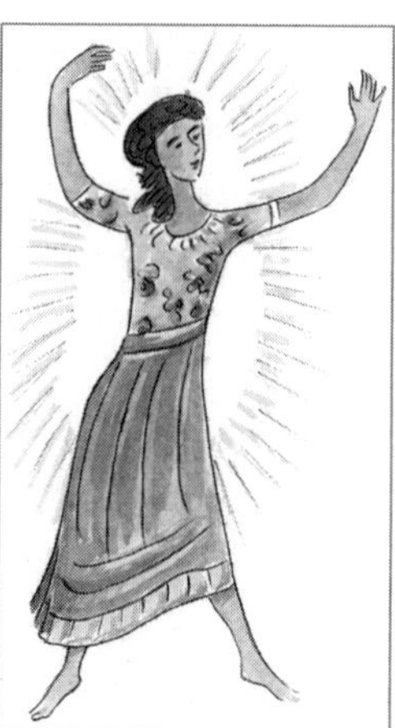

Heavenly Joy responds:

"Oh, you are blind and deaf; you don't know what you're saying. God created a radiant human being but because of our unfaithfulness, snakes lead us into the sea of misery. Yet behold the sun, the moon, and the stars and all the glory and beauty on earth and contemplate the blessings God bestowed on humankind. Do you see that the same human in all of her rashness forgets God?

"You are basically a charlatan and a cheat, abominable, immoral, and perverted. Instead of trust you cultivate only the diabolical—you don't want to know anything and you don't realize where God's cure for you lies. Who, if not God, gives you all the lustrous, splendid gifts of life? When day rushes your way, you call it night, and when good fortune crosses your path, it is misfortune to you. When you are doing well, you claim you are doing badly. Hence, you are the site of the darkness, of the doomed.

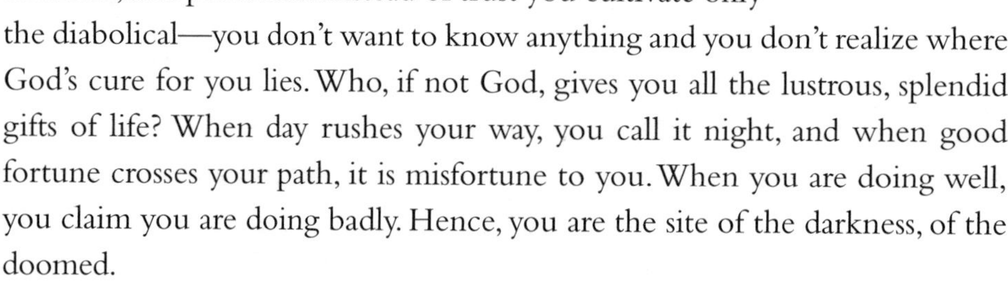

"I, however, have heaven on earth today because I perceive everything God has created. You call this universe a misfortune. I tenderly hold close to my heart the blossoming roses, the lilies, and all the green freshness of life and praise God's works while you accumulate pain. You are woeful in all your deeds. You are nothing short of the evil spirits who negate God in all their actions. I do things differently. I present all my doings to God, as even in sadness there still lies joy and joy contains happiness, so that it does not alternate like day and night" (LVM).

Heavenly Joy

Heavenly joy reigns in companionship with God. All people have an (ab)original yearning for the "kiss of God" and the embrace of their Creator, because he has poured this tender love inside all creation.

Organ Relationship

Melancholy, Weltschmerz, sadness, misery, distress, anguish, depression, pain and suffering, and black bile relate to the malfunction of the central nervous system and a lack in happy-making neurotransmitters like serotonins and endorphins. The skull protects this center and counts as the first vertebrae. This finding relates back to research by the poet Johann Wolfgang von Goethe, the first to understand the anatomy of the vertebrae.

Melancholy and madness, the enemies of our physical and psychic immunity, attack joy and happiness. There are times when every one of us is overshadowed by negative forces that are virulent. The virus of melancholy and depression invades our souls and attacks with great power. The emotional problem is transferred to our bodies, causing a biochemical chain reaction that is primarily responsible for almost all autoaggressive sicknesses, like heart attack, stroke, cancer, polyarthritis, neurodermitis, and fibromyalgia, to name just a few of the approximately 40,000 aggression illnesses of today. Most of these diseases are chronic and therefore "incurable" by conventional medicine because the evoking spiritual risk factors are seriously neglected. In her vision Hildegard sees a dry desert, darkness, and attacking worms—all symbols for autoaggressive ailments (LVM).

Origin of Sadness

Shortly after World War II an economic miracle *(Wirtschaftswunder)* began. It offered food and prosperity for everybody after a period of starvation and misery. But surprisingly enough, the abundance of material goods caused quite the opposite: sadness and depression. What people really were looking for was to satisfy their hunger for spirituality. After fifty years of war and terror, spirituality was gone. God was "dead" in the mind of the public.
Hildegard writes:

> I caught sight of still other spirits and heard them roar, Who is God, whom I abhor? These spirits lure men and women into Weltschmerz, so they wither away in sorrow and experience life as suffering.

Hildegard of Bingen sees depression, psychosis, suicide, and anxiety as a consequence of this godlessness. And godlessness in our modern culture often causes people to resort to antidepressants, narcotics, and tranquilizers in order to suppress their world-weariness.

Our civilized society cultivates sadness by forgetting and disregarding God and ceasing to appreciate the Creation. Today we worship other idols and icons: political figures, corporate executives, and celebrities, all of whom captivate us with their status and fame. And so sadness and depression have become a mass sickness of our times, a psychosis. Humankind can restore happiness only by remembering and recognizing the image of God again amid this field of rubble.

Against Melancholy

Since the Garden of Eden, people do not live in unblemished heavenly joy anymore. From then on black bile has overflowed at any sign of worry or concern, and we may become slaves to pathogenic passions like sorrow, anger, rage, frustration, irritation, and finally Melancholy. Under such circumstances Hildegard recommends a whole string of remedies capable of neutralizing black bile and strengthening the joy-bringing healing process.

"If the human being did not possess the bitterness of the gallbladder and the darkness of the bile," writes Hildegard in her pharmacology, "she would be perpetually happy." Therefore, the path out of sadness simultaneously leads to health. This is the reason that depression must be professionally treated and not masked by antidepressants. Everything healthy, healing, and beautiful contains an impact that brings joy, be it in the form of the scent of roses or lilies, a precious stone, or what is known as the *anti-melancholica*, which neutralize black bile and stabilize the nerves. Hildegard's anti-melancholica improve the complexion, lending some color to the customarily pale skin tone of those who are depressed.

SPELT, PSYLLIUM SEEDS, AND PELLITORY *(ANACYCLUS PYRETHRUM)*

The primary treatment in Hildegard's medicine is spelt (or durum); he who eats spelt obtains a cheerful spirit, and his black bile—the cause of all serious disease—is eradicated. It is advisable to start the day with a breakfast of cooked spelt cereal. In fact, the very best treatment, nutritionally speaking, is to substitute spelt for all wheat and wheat products.

Psyllium seeds (the seeds of plantain or ribwort) are another excellent anti-melancholica. "They gladden the individual's depressed disposition by virtue of their sweet temperament," writes Hildegard. Sprinkling a teaspoon of psyllium seeds over every meal will ensure optimum digestion. The psyllium seeds remove black bile, poisonous substances, and waste products from the intestines, providing an excellent purification of the bloodstream, a prerequisite for good circulation of the blood.

Pellitory is a panacea; sprinkle 2 or 3 teaspoons over any food, or add it while cooking. "By reducing the harmful substances in the blood and increasing the 'good blood,' pellitory produces a clear mind," writes Hildegard. It supplies the weak with new vitality, even when their physical strength is failing. Pellitory promotes good digestion and does not permit anything to leave the body undigested. Pellitory is a universal remedy for both the healthy and the sick because it sustains health and expels disease from the body."

NOURISHMENT FOR THE NERVES

Normally the privilege of youth, good nerves are the result of the flawless interplay among all five senses: sharp eyes, fine hearing, a keen sense of smell, a delicate sense of taste, and a sensitive sense of touch. Nerve cookies invigorate all five senses and prevent them from dulling with age. They generate a merry disposition, optimism, and a joyous heart, and strengthen the nerves. This effect is attributed to nutmeg, which is notorious for its psychotropic properties and its stimulating effect on the nerves. Nerve cookies, or intelligence cookies, have proved reliable and successful in the treatment of schoolchildren with difficulties in concentrating. In this case, 3 to 5 cookies a day are adequate for an effective treatment.

Spice Cookies for the Nerves

These cookies not only remove all bitterness from the heart, but they also sharpen intelligence and enhance all five senses.

1 1/2 cups butter
3 cups brown sugar
2 eggs
1/2 tsp. salt
2 1/2 tsp. cinnamon
2 1/2 tsp. nutmeg
1/2 tsp. cloves
1 cup grated almonds
4 tsp. baking powder
6 cups spelt flour

Cream the butter and brown sugar until fluffy. Add the eggs and beat well. Add remaining ingredients and knead thoroughly to combine, then roll into a log. Wrap in baking paper and refrigerate. Once the dough has hardened (about 2 hours), preheat the oven to 375°F. Cut dough into 1/4-inch slices and bake on a lightly greased cookie sheet 10 to 12 minutes, until cookies are golden.

Adults can eat 4 or 5 cookies daily; children should eat no more than 3, lest they become too smart!

SARDONYX, ONYX, AND CHALCEDONY

Three stones induce strengthening of the senses.

The **sardonyx,** a precious stone, must be worn on the bare skin or licked often in order to enhance all five senses.

"If a person carries the sardonyx on her bare skin," writes Hildegard, "and in addition places it in her mouth so that her breath touches it, removes it, and places it inside her mouth again, then her intellect, knowledge, and all her sensory perceptions will be strengthened. In this manner all excessive anger, futility, and lack of discipline are withdrawn from the person. Because of the intense purity of the sardonyx, the devil hates and flees it."

The **onyx** alleviates both reactive sadness and the sadness that results from serious sickness: "When you are weighed down by melancholy, examine the onyx intensely, then place it in your mouth immediately and the depressed mood will leave you," writes Hildegard.

The beautiful bluish **chalcedony** stone, worn on the skin as either a necklace or a bracelet, is another aid for the senses: "This precious stone has the energy to avert all ailing from the bearer, lending her a peaceful attitude unshakable by anger," writes Hildegard. "Her demeanor will become so good-natured that there is hardly a person who could provoke her through injustice and ignite her temper, not even if it were justified."

One can often recognize friends of Hildegard by virtue of the chalcedony, which has saved many of them from the depths of sadness. The stone is worn as a necklace over the so-called anger vein or as a bracelet around the wrist on top of the "pulse artery."

SWEET ALMONDS AND OATS

Sweet almonds, eaten often, provide excellent nourishment for the nerves, for they replenish the empty brain and promote a healthy complexion. A drained brain and an unhealthy complexion are a result of disturbed body fat and protein metabolism. In addition, sweet almonds contain high-quality protein for the "metabolism" of the nerves.

For healthy individuals, oats eaten for breakfast in the form of flakes, porridge, or grits are almost as good as spelt. Writes Hildegard, "Oats notably stimulate the taste buds and the sense of smell. For healthy individuals, oatmeal provides enjoyment and sustains health; it promotes a sunny disposition and a pure and bright openness. Their skin becomes beautiful and their flesh robust and healthy."

Oats are not suited for consumption by the sick, however, as they require good circulation of the digestive system: "If a sick person were to eat oatmeal, it would coagulate inside the stomach and cause a mucous catarrh, because oats cool down the body too much."

FENNEL, SAVORY, AND HYSSOP

Eating **fennel** eliminates another characteristic of melancholy—bad body odor.

"Eaten in any form," writes Hildegard, "fennel brings humans a sense of joyfulness and endows them with a beautiful complexion, pleasant body odor, and excellent digestion."

Fennel is healthy in any form—in a tea, as a vegetable, or, even better, in fennel tablets, with 3 tablets taken 3 times daily, before each meal. Individuals who suffer from heartburn take an additional 3 pills after every meal. This not only rids the body of black bile, but also neutralizes the acidity of the gallbladder.

Savory gladdens the heart, and a weak heart can also be the cause of sadness. It is unclear, however, whether sadness weakens the heart or a weak heart causes sadness. If the heart is afflicted, Hildegard recommends savory:

"If a person has acquired a weak heart and a sick stomach, he should eat this fresh herb and it will provide new strength. Individuals with a depressed nature are gladdened by eating savory. Eating this herb also cures and clears up the eyes."

Savory is the best herb for old age; it has proved immensely effective in the treatment of both a frail heart and stomach as well as dulled eyesight (cataracts).

Hyssop is an extraordinary remedy containing powers that provide happiness. Hildegard writes:

"If a person's liver has become sick from sadness, he shall cook chicken with hyssop before the sickness runs rampant, and eat this chicken together with the hyssop often. He should also eat fresh hyssop marinated in wine and drink the wine too. For such a disease [melancholy], hyssop is even more beneficial than for someone afflicted only by lung problems."

QUENCHED WINE: THE BEST ANTIDOTE

Quenched wine is Hildegard's best and easiest treatment for melancholy. It strengthens the nerves and banishes anxiety and anger reliably and swiftly. Fifty percent of all nerve complaints are directly caused by anger—our own, our partner's, our spouse's, our mother-in-law's. Fury and anger cause the gallbladder to overflow and lead to an autogenic poisoning of the blood with black bile.

One can even drink quenched wine in the morning, after getting up "on the wrong side of the bed." To salvage such a day, combat it by drinking the warm quenched wine prior to all other activities. If that is not enough, and it is feasible, prepare a large quantity of quenched wine and take it to work in a thermos bottle. That may just save your day.

The black bile must be eradicated; otherwise, it may manifest itself in severe illnesses or mood swings, because, writes Hildegard, anger can lead to violence and sadness causes disease: "If a person is spurred to anger or melancholy, she should quickly heat up some wine to the boiling point, quench it with a little cold water, and drink it while warm. In this way, the substance [black bile], which has led to the eruption of anger, is neutralized."

Quenched Wine

Bring half a glass of the best wine (white or red) to a boil. As soon as bubbles start to form, add a shot of cold water, remove the wine from the heat, and drink it while warm in small sips. When the entire family is angry with one another, quenched wine promptly restores peace in the home. The effect is dependent neither on the amount nor the content of alcohol in the quenched wine because, as a result of the boiling, the alcohol evaporates as it simmers at a temperature as low as 176°F. Children or people sensitive to wine and alcohol receive only a shot glass or a few spoonfuls.

ARUM FOR DEPRESSION

In the case of severe depression—that is, melancholy that lasts for months and months, Hildegard recommends arum tonic:

"Anyone who has a fever in his stomach, which can result in a shivering fit, shall simmer arum root in wine, let it cool, and then submerge a hot metal [immersion heater] into this wine to reheat it and drink it while warm. The wine will take away the mucus and the fever in the same way that fire melts snow. Everyone who suffers from melancholy has a gloomy disposition and is perpetually depressed. Such individuals should drink the arum tonic often, and it will diminish their depression as well as the fever."

VIOLET ELIXIR, COWSLIP, AND RUE

For sadness in connection with a lung condition, Hildegard recommends violet elixir:

"Anyone who is weighed down by melancholy and anger, which cause damage to the lungs, should cook violets in wine, strain the liquid through a cloth, and add as much galangal and licorice as desired. Reheat the wine, clarify the beverage, and drink it. It will suppress melancholy, cheer the spirit, and heal the lungs."

In an ailment of the lungs (without a classical infection) as a result of the flu or a cold that will not improve, there are two main causes: either an older liver damage (jaundice or hepatitis) or a mood infirmity. If the liver is affected, the remedy is hart's-tongue fern elixir; the treatment for melancholy is the violet elixir.

Violet Elixir

The violet elixir aids in the remedy of early-menopause depression with an affliction of the lungs and chronic despair, as well as moderate melancholy and apathy, with or without an affliction of the lungs.

1 1/2 teaspoons violet leaves and flowers
1 liter wine
2 teaspoons licorice
1 teaspoon galangal

Boil the violet leaves and flowers in the wine. Remove from heat, then add the licorice and the galangal. Let stand overnight, then bring to a boil again and strain. Drink half a cup a day for 4 to 6 weeks.

Take a break from the treatment and possibly reinstate it, until a distinct positive mood alteration occurs; when the violet elixir does not taste good anymore, it is a sure indication of the revival of the spirit of life.

In springtime, cowslip elixir helps the depressed to "unlock the gates of heaven" once again.

Pick a big bouquet of cowslips, tie them into a compress, and bind it across the heart overnight. If a friend picks these flowers for someone she loves, the effect of the treatment is doubled.

For heartburn, Hildegard recommends completing every meal with bitter herbs. One herb always to keep on hand (whether in your own herb garden, in potted plants on the window sill, or from an herbal store) is rue, for it alleviates black bile. Rue eases the improper heat and cold of melancholy: "the melancholic person will feel better by ending her meals with some rue. Even when the meal itself invokes pain, eating rue after the meal will lessen that reaction." Periodically eating a few fresh leaves of rue after meals gets rid not only of melancholy, but also of the nuisance of subsequent heartburn.

Spiritual Healing

Divine joy yearns to open the melancholic's eyes to the the cosmos, to Creation, to the sun, the moon, the stars. Negative thinking attracts more negativity, and forever looking on the dark side of life will fulfill its own prophecy. Heavenly joy beholds the blooming roses, lilies, and the greening vitality of life and recognizes God in all creation.

Psalms 104 and 105 declare the celebration and festivity filled with the exuberance of divine joy.

Chapter 8

Fasting: Discover Your Real Personality

Hildegard fasting is a spiritual journey to discover the real personality with its thirty-five virtues. We can reach this goal by three different fasting methods: long-term fasting, bread fasting, and hard-core fasting.

Long-term Fasting

First is the easy long-term fasting, with powerful foods for the mind based on spelt, fruits, and vegetables. This method has been successful for everybody, the healthy and the sick, especially for all overweight people who want to lose some pounds and feel better. The best food for a long-term reduction diet is also preventative and heals modern civilization's killer sicknesses like coronary heart disease, stroke, cancer, arteriosclerosis, and diabetes. The basis is not vitamins, supplements, and/or calories but rather the healing forces hidden in our nutrition. Hildegard describes an abundance of food as medicine that heals both body and soul and sustains life.

The best food for a harmonic balance of body and soul is based on the mild digestible complex carbohydrates found in grains, vegetables, nuts, and fruits. At the top of the list is spelt, an old unhybridized grain that contains everything we need including proteins, complex carbohydrates, unsaturated fats, and especially all forty-five minerals and trace minerals necessary to build and regenerate cartilage and bone. The abundance of minerals neutralizes a stressful lifestyle, which produces too much gallic acid and causes inflammation and autoaggression. Spelt contains an essential substance—thiocyanate, or rhodanide—that occurs in tear fluid, nose secretion, blood, and especially mother's milk, to stimulate the immune system in the newborn baby.

Thiocyanate has fundamental effects on our health, as it stimulates the red marrow in our bones to produce enough healthy blood and to make the cell membranes impenetrable to cancer-causing viruses.

The physiological effects of thiocyanate in spelt have been intensively studied by Professor Wolfgang Weuffen, at the University of Greifswald in Germany. Following are some of his findings.

Thiocyanate in spelt, fruits, and vegetables:

- stimulates proliferation of all growing cells including skin, hair, and fingernails
- stimulates bone marrow to produce cells for the blood and immune system, as well as sex cells in both men and women
- is active against all kinds of inflammation
- is protective against viral, bacterial, and fungal infections
- guards against disease damage through heredity (genes) and during pregnancy
- is antitoxic
- is antiallergenic

Spelt contains no stress-related, allergy-related proteins, as wheat does. The new scientific findings are excellent support for and proof of Hildegard's visionary discoveries about spelt. She writes:

"Spelt is the very best grain—warming, lubricating, and of high nutritional value. It is better tolerated by the body than any other grain. Spelt provides its consumer with good muscle flesh and good blood and confers a cheerful disposition. It provides a happy mind and a joyful spirit. No matter how you eat spelt, either as a bread or in cooked food, it is tasty and easy to digest."

To my knowledge, this is the first time people have been treated and healed systematically with spelt. Critical examination proves these successes are due 90 percent to the change in diet from wheat to spelt. Healing results are possible only with 100 percent organically grown spelt, free from the harmful pesticides, chemicals, food additives, and environmental pollutants found in all other conventionally grown grain.

The best recommendation is spelt 3 times a day:

Breakfast: hot spelt cereal, cream of spelt, waffles, pancakes, spelt muffins, spelt bread, spelt coffee
Lunch: spelt soup, spelt sandwich, spelt sprinkled on salad, spelt burgers
Dinner: spelt rice, spelt pasta, vegetables, salad with spelt kernels, and fruit desserts

Kitchen spices such as pelletory, galangal, thyme, cooked onion, raw garlic, parsley, nutmeg, salt, and pepper are a healthful part of your diet.

Vegetables should be cooked: fennel, chestnuts, beets, carrots, pumpkin, all kinds of beans including organic soybeans, celery, or chickpeas in the form of falafel or hummus.

Use sunflower, walnut, and almond oil for cooking and dressings.

Avoid strawberries, peaches, plums, and leeks, which cause bad blood, inflammations, and eczema as well as a weakening of the immune system.

For beverages, drink fennel tea, spelt coffee, herbal tea, green tea, and fruit juice.

BREAD FASTING

The three- to nine-month bread-fasting diet is for all people who want to lose weight slowly and reliably. This mild diet allows normal food, as listed above, and every second day only spelt bread, fennel tea, and green salad, with as many spelt kernels as desired.

There are no feelings of hunger or thirst. Avoid cheese, meat, and eggs, other than perhaps once a week, and enjoy more fish, lamb, and chicken without skin.

HARD-CORE FASTING

This is generally recommended for just one week and then an additional regeneration week. Under the guidance of a Hildegard fasting master, this is the universal healing remedy for twenty-eight spiritual risk factors, but not for the following seven negative risk factors, which are excluded from fasting:

- No. 1: Love of the material world
- No. 13: Unhappiness
- No. 14: Immoderation
- No. 15: Doom
- No. 16: Arrogance
- No. 26: Instability, inconstancy
- No. 35: Melancholy, depression

Note: Sick people who have lost weight should not fast but instead should be regenerated. People with acute illnesses such as epilepsy, multiple sclerosis, stroke, heart attack, ataxia, and convulsions are excluded from fasting.

Begin fasting in a group under the supervision of an expert for no longer than ten days at a time. Therapeutic fasting for longer periods must be done in a clinic. It is best to start with two or three days of preparation, eating only spelt rice, vegetables, fresh fruit, and salad. Tobacco, coffee, and alcohol, as well as unnecessary drugs, are completely withdrawn. This is also the best way to quit smoking and drinking. Consult your doctor for advice.

Hildegard fasting is based on abstinence from eating but drinking herbal tea, spelt coffee, fruit and vegetable juices, and lots of spring- or well water, a minimum of three quarts a day. Your body will need plenty of exercise and *viriditas* from all four elements—fresh air, water, sunshine, and earth—enjoyed through walks or even mountain climbing. You may be surprised that after three days you feel strong and vital, with clarity of thought and even creativity. Fasting requires its own rules. Retreat from your daily routine—stay in peaceful surroundings, with people who have supportive interests, and with no telephone in sight!

Vegetable-Spelt Broth

People will not experience hunger during fasting if they cook a fasting soup based on spelt and lots of vegetables.

To 1 cup of spelt per person, add 3 cups of water, some chopped carrots, beans, beets, celery, and herbs to taste. Boil for twenty to thirty minutes. Strain, discarding the solids, and drink only the liquid. Enjoy a cup of fasting soup once a day. It contains all the vital vitamins and minerals you'll need.

PURGING AND CLEANSING

A beneficial side effect of fasting is the release of poisons and waste products from both in the tissues and throughout the body. Fasting begins with an effective colon cleansing—no colon hydrotherapy, which is much too strong. Hildegard suggests a purgative cookie made from a mixture of spices—ginger, sweet wood licorice, and euphorbia.

"Before eating this cookie," writes Hildegard, "warm yourself in front of a fire if it is cold outside, and afterward rest on your bed while remaining awake. Then, walk slowly and do not let the cold overwhelm you. In this way the spices retain the good fluids, whereas the noxious *(noxi humores)* ones will leave the body."

You can also begin your fast without the purgative by administering a double enema. Use 1 pint of fennel or chamomile tea water, hold it in, and release in 5 minutes. Repeat the same procedure with 2 pints and continue doing this daily before you go to bed. Enemas are essential during fasting, as toxic wastes would otherwise remain in the body and be reabsorbed into the blood.

Fasting effectively stimulates the building and growth of new cells, restoring health and rejuvenating the body. After the first three days, the body will nurture itself. When nutrition is required, it will burn and digest from its own inner storehouse. First attended are those cells and tissues that are dead, diseased, or damaged, such as tumorous cells, arterial sclerotic plaques, and rubbish in body and mind. This accelerates the force of regeneration. The level of blood cholesterol and blood pressure will return to normal.

During fasting a vast amount of toxins and wastes (uric acids) leave the body and in so doing retoxify the blood for a very short time. Sometimes those who fast experience a crisis: Retoxification may cause headache, pain, dizziness, or weakness. These ailments during the time of fasting can all be effectively treated with Hildegard's remedies.

Parsley-Honey Wine

This heart wine, taken as needed during fasting, has been shown to normalize both high and low blood pressure.

1 liter red wine
10 big sprigs of parsley
2 tablespoons wine vinegar
150 grams good-quality honey

To the red wine add the parsley and wine vinegar and boil for 5 minutes. Add the honey and boil once more, remove foam, and refill in the original wine bottle.

Take 1 to 3 shot glasses of wine in cases of weakness, dizziness, heart pain, or bad circulation.

GALANGAL TABLETS

The emergency drug galangal immediately lowers high blood pressure, improves impaired circulation, and prevents heart attack.

FENNEL TABLETS

A few "happy-making" fennel tablets promote good breath and clear vision.

FASTING SCHEDULE

7:00 A.M.: Wake up with dry brush massage; take a hot shower, then a cold one.
7:30 A.M.: Exercise; gymnastics
8:00 A.M.: Herb tea or spelt coffee
12:00 NOON: Hot fasting soup

12:30 P.M.:	Rest with a warm liver compress (a hot-water bottle or towel on the liver area)
3:00 P.M.:	Extended walk or hiking
6:00 P.M.:	Fruit juice (apple with cinnamon, for example) and warm fennel tea
8:00 P.M.:	Meditation, singing, playing, reading
10:00 P.M.:	Enema, warm shower, and rest

REGENERATION WEEK

Break the fast with a baked apple on the evening before the new week starts.

Breakfast

Spelt rice or hot spelt cereal. Add 1/2 cup of spelt (may be coarsely ground, which takes less time to cook) to 1 cup of water and simmer for 20 to 30 minutes. Spice with cinnamon, galangal, pellitory *(Anacyclus pyrethrum),* and honey.

Eat and chew slowly; never overeat. Tastes excellent with cooked apple slices.

Noon Meal

Vegetable soup and salad. Place fresh chopped garden lettuce in a bowl. Add 3 spoonfuls of spelt kernels and dress with sunflower oil, wine vinegar, and some brown sugar.

Supper

Spelt bread. Mix together 1 pound of whole-grain spelt flour, 3 teaspoons of spice (thyme, galangal, and pellitory), a large pinch of salt, 1/2 package of yeast, and 1 pint of warm water.

Knead the dough. Leave it to rise for 1 1/2 hours, then bake in a hot oven for 1 hour. Make a spread from vegetables or out of cottage cheese with herbs or fresh cheese spiced with cumin.

Repeat these menus for one week in order to regain a perfectly normal digestion without the aid of laxatives. In order to continue the benefits, maintain the Hildegard diet and exercise positive spiritual values. This is a great way to prevent diseases and degeneration of the body. It improves nerves and mental functioning, normalizes body and brain chemistry, lowers blood cholesterol, and flushes out toxins. At the end of the fast, one feels like a new person.

The virtues stamp us with an indelible stamp and remind us that we are "sons of God" (Romans 8:14–17).

And in the words of Colossians 3:12–17, "Therefore as God's chosen people, holy and dearly loved, clothe yourselves with compassion, kindness, humility, gentleness, and patience. Bear with each other and forgive whatever grievances you may have against one another. Forgive as the Lord forgave you. And over all these virtues put love, which binds them all in perfect unity.

"Let the peace of Christ rule in your hearts, since as members of one body you were called to peace. And be thankful. Let the word of Christ dwell in you richly as you teach and admonish one another with all wisdom, and as you sing psalms, hymns, and spiritual songs with gratitude in your hearts to God. And whatever you do, whether in word or deed, do it all in the name of the Lord Jesus, giving thanks to God the Father through him."

Bibliography

Original Latin books of Hildegard of Bingen

Carmina Sanctae Hildegardis. Edited by Pudentiana Bart, OSB, et al. Salzburg: Otto Müller Verlag, 1969.

Causae et Curae (CC). Edited by Paul Kaiser. Leipzig: Teubner Verlag, 1903.

Hildegardis Scivias (SC). Corpus Christianorum. Brepols: Turnhout, 1978.

Liber Divinorum Operum (LDO). Corpus Christianorum. Brepols: Turnhout, 1996.

Liber Vitae Meritorum (LVM). Corpus Christianorum. Brepols: Turnhout, 1995.

Opera Omnia S. Hildegardis (Physica). Edited by Jaques Paul Migne. Paris, 1882.

English Editions

Fox, Matthew. *Illuminations of Hildegard of Bingen.* Santa Fe: Bear & Company, 1985.

Hozeski, Bruce, trans. *Scivias.* Santa Fe: Bear & Company, 1986.

Strehlow, Dr. Wighard, and Hertzka, Dr. Gottfried. *Hildegard of Bingen's Medicine.* Santa Fe: Bear & Company, 1989.

Index

abortion, 114–115
abstinence, as virtue, 3, 40, 108–111
acid, 110–111
  of blood, 113
active daily life, 132
agate, as healing stone, 225
addictions, 86, 199–200
allergies
  to chemicals, 85
  to food, 91, 102, 106
  and spelt, 245–246
almonds, sweet, 239
amethyst, as healing stone, 11, 89, 139, 143, 188, 219, 230
amor caritatis, 61, 143, 164
angels, 50–51
  as healers, 45–48
anger, as vice, 3, 40, 92–103
anima, 59
animal
  skin as clothing, 84
  spirit keepers, 36
anti-melancholica, 236–237
aquamarine, as healing stone, 203–204
archetypes, 44
aromatherapy, 76–77. *See also* smell
arrogance, as vice, 4, 40, 139–142
arum, 241
audio-vision, 63–64
autoaggressive sicknesses, xii, 3–7, 15–17, 85, 92
  and black bile, 97, 99, 215
  curing of, 100–103
  and fasting, 245
  risk factors for, 155, 191, 196, 201
autonomic nervous system, 55
avarice, as vice, 7, 40, 225–230

balance. *See* harmony
beryl, 203–204
bitterness of heart, as vice, 3, 40
biophoton energy, 23, 27–28, 30
bitterness of heart, 111–115, 238
black bile, 83, 93, 97–99, 106, 112, 215, 231, 235, 236, 237
  and fennel, 240
  and quenched wine, 241
blessedness
  as virtue, 4, 40, 124–128
bloodletting, 131
body
  and soul, relationship between, 22, 24–33, 53–55, 58–59
  systems and central nervous system, 55–58
body odor, 240
brain waves, 69–70
bread fasting, 246
burying the dead, 86

cataracts, 240
central nervous system. *See* nervous system
chalcedony, 92, 112, 239
charity, 148
  as virtue, 4, 40, 142–147
chastity, as virtue, 5, 40, 164–167
chemicals
  in buildings, 85
  in clothing, 84
cherubim, role of, in healing, 49–50
childbirth and salvation, 135
childhood virtues, 137–139
children and their fathers, 29
Christ, 158–159
cloister, Hildegard's, 53–54
clothes, natural, and compassion, 84
compassion, seven deeds of, 82–87
compassion, as virtue, 3, 40, 79–88
conception, 135–136
concern for worldly goods, as vice, 6, 40, 188–192
concord, as virtue, 7, 40, 203–207
contention, as vice, 4, 40, 121–124
Contractus, Hermanus, 177–178
cosmic Christ, 51, 53
cosmic psychosynthesis, 23
cowardice, as vice, 3, 40, 88–92
cowslip, 242
craving, as vice, 6, 40, 197–203
crystal therapy for
  anger, 92
  arrogance, 139
  avarice, 225
  bitterness of heart, 112
  concern for worldly goods, 188
  contention, 121
  cowardice, 89
  craving, 197
  despair, 160
  discord, 203–204
  disobedience, 153
  envy, 143
  gluttony, 108
  hard-heartedness, 80

immoderation, 128–129
inappropriate mirth, 104
injustice, 169
instability, 185
lack of faith, 156
lethargy, 175
lost soul, 133
love of entertainment, 74
lying, 118
material love, 62
melancholy, 230
oblivion, 179
obscenity, 164
obstinacy, 192
occultism, 219
petulance, 69
scurrility, 213
thirst for glory, 149–150
unhappiness, 124
vagabondage, 216
wickedness, 115
crystal water, 11, 104
crystals and stones, healing power of, 9–11, 28.

DNA, 27, 28, 30, 147
dedication to God, as virtue, 7, 40, 219–223
deodorant, 76
depression, 76, 98, 99, 231
menopausal, 242
despair, as vice, 160–163
desperation, as vice, 5, 40
devotion, as virtue, 4, 40, 115–117
diamond, as healing stone, 108, 118
diamond water, 80
diet, 102, 217
during fasting, 248, 249
discipline, as virtue, 3, 40, 69–74
discord, as vice, 7, 40, 203–207
discretion, as virtue, 4, 40, 128–133
disobedience, as vice, 5, 40, 153–155
doom, as vice, 4, 40
drinking, fasting to quit, 247
drugs. *See* medications

ears, 69–70
inner, 63–64
role of, in healing, 48–49
earth, sound of, 147–148
eating. *See* diet *and* fasting
ecological housing, and compassion, 85
emerald, as healing stone, 11, 115, 124, 133, 149, 175
enema, during fasting, 248
energy. *See* life energy
environment, collapse of, 34
envy, as vice, 5, 40, 142–147
evil, origins of, 93
eyes
inner, 63–64
role of, in healing, 48, 49–50
as window of soul, 62–63

faith, as virtue, 5, 40, 156–160
fasting, 244–251. *See also* Healing *for individual vices*
bread, 246
to find God, 179
hard-core, 247–251
long-term, 244–246
to manage anger, 96
not recommended, 139–140, 142, 149, 163, 187, 247
for self-analysis, 43–44
feet, virtues and weaknesses, 212–243
feng shui, 204
fennel, 76, 240, 249
Fennel Eye Remedy, 76
Fennel Tea, 76
fireballs, 25–27, 34
five forces, 183–184
five senses, 237, 238
food. *See also* diet
and compassion, 83
and healthy skin, 91
forgiveness, 229–230
fortitude, as virtue, 6, 40, 174–178
four
elements and four humors, 12–15
number, significance of, 13, 18–20, 25
rhythms, 70

galangal, 193, 246, 249, 250
generosity, as virtue, 3, 40, 111–115
gluttony, as vice, 3, 40, 108–111
God, 158
godlessness, 236
God's army, 51
God's victory, as virtue, 3, 40, 88–92
gold cure, 92
Gold Topaz Prayer, 32, 179, 224
gold topaz
as healing stone, 121, 179, 213, 222
wine, 62
Golden Mean, 130
golden rules of Hildegard, 73–74
Golden Tent, 32–33
Good as Gold, 93
green energy. See *viriditas*

happiness. *See* heavenly joy
hard-heartedness, as vice, 3, 40, 79–88
harmony, 184
of body and soul, 42, 204–205
and fasting, 244–245
and music, 27, 72–73, 147
with nature in healing, 86
as a right, 198
in the universe, 17, 24, 25, 37, 69, 147–148, 153

healing, 44–45
  and anger, 103
  and arrogance, 142
  and avarice, 229–230
  and bitterness of heart, 115
  and concern for worldly goods, 192
  and contention, 123
  and cowardice, 92
  craving, 203
  and crystals and stones, 9–11, 28
  and despair, 163
  and discord, 207
  and disobedience, 155
  without drugs, 86
  and envy, 149
  and fasting, 244
  and four humors, 13
  four stages of, 182
  and gluttony, 111
  and hard-heartedness, 88
  and immoderation, 132
  and injustice, 174
  and instability, 187
  and lack of faith, 160
  and lethargy, 178
  and lost soul, 136
  and love of entertainment, 79
  and lying, 121
  and melancholy, 243
  and music, 72
  and oblivion, 182, 184
  and obscenity, 167
  and obstinacy, 197
  and occultism, 223
  and petulance,73–74
  and scurrility, 215
  and spirituality, 18, 68–69
  and thirst for glory, 152
  and unhappiness, 128
  and vagabondage, 218
  by virtues, 41–43, 58–59
  with vortex energy, 152
  and wickedness, 117
heavenly desire, as virtue, 6, 40, 188–192
heavenly joy, as virtue, 7, 40, 230–243
heavenly love, as virtue, 3, 40, 62–68
high-voltage wires, 85
holiness, as virtue, 6, 40, 178–184
Holy Spirit, 159
hope, as virtue, 5, 40, 160–163
housing, and compassion, 85
humility, as virtue, 4, 40, 139–142
humoral pathology, 12
hyssop, 240

immoderation, as vice, 4, 40, 128–133
inappropriate mirth, as vice, 3, 40, 103–106
infancy, 137–138
injustice, as vice, 6, 40, 169–174
instability, as vice, 6, 40, 185–188
intelligence, 238

jasper, as healing stone, 69, 74, 128, 185, 192, 193, 216
joy. *See* heavenly joy
Jung, Carl Gustav, 44, 202
justice, as virtue, 6, 40, 169–174

lack of faith, as vice, 5, 40, 156–160
lavender, 75
Law of Divine Compassion, 81
leaky-gut syndrome, 97–101, 215
lethargy, as vice, 6, 40, 174–178
letting go, as virtue, 6, 40, 197–203
Lex Divina, 81
life of contemplation, 132
life energy, 23–24, 25–28, 33
  fasting as source of, 44
Lily Oil, 75
lost soul, as vice, 133–136
love of entertainment, as vice, 3, 40, 74–79
love of simplicity, as virtue, 3, 40, 74–79
lucida materia, 204
lung conditions, 242
lying, as vice, 4, 40, 117–121

material love, as vice, 3, 40, 62–68
mathematics and music, 73
medications, 236
  and compassion, 83–84
  and suicide, 231
melancholy
  and acid, 110
  as vice, 7, 40, 230–243
men and children they father, 29
menopausal depression, 242
microflora, 99–100
Militia Dei, 51
money and material love, 65
moon, 36–37. *See also* planets
music
  and healing, 72
  and mathematics, 73

nerves, 237–238
nervous system, 42, 55–58
Nicene Creed, 33, 158, 159
nutmeg, as antidepressant, 237
nutrition. *See* diet *and* food

oats, 239
obedience, as virtue, 5, 40, 153–155
oblivion, as vice, 6, 40, 178–184
obscenity, as vice, 5, 40, 164–167
obstinacy, as vice, 6, 40, 192–197
occultism, as vice, 7, 40, 219–223
olivine, 169

onyx
  as healing stone, 230, 239
  wine, 104
Ordo Virtutum, 58
organ relationship with
  anger, 103
  arrogance, 141
  avarice, 228–229
  bitterness of heart, 113–114
  concern for worldly goods, 191
  contention, 123
  cowardice, 90
  craving, 201
  despair, 163
  discord, 206–207
  disobedience, 155
  envy, 146
  gluttony, 111
  hard-heartedness, 87
  immoderation, 131
  inappropriate mirth, 105
  injustice, 173
  instability, 187
  lack of faith, 159–160
  lethargy, 177
  lost soul, 134–135
  love of entertainment, 79
  lying, 120–121
  material love, 67
  melancholy, 235
  oblivion, 182
  obscenity, 167
  obstinacy, 195–196
  occultism, 221
  petulance, 72
  scurrility, 214–215
  thirst for glory, 151–152
  unhappiness, 126
  vagabondage, 217
  wickedness, 117
organs
  and four humors, 13–15
  and virtues and vices, 3–7
overweight people and fasting, 244

Parsley-Honey Wine, 106, 249
patience, 95
peace, as virtue, 4, 121–124
Pear Honey, 101–102
pellitory, 237, 246, 250
peridot, as healing stone, 169
pessimism. *See* melancholy
petulance, as vice, 3, 40, 69–74
planets, 22, 36–37
power center of the soul, 183–184
Prayer, Gold Topaz, 32, 179, 224
pregnancy, 135–136
  and health of baby, 42–43, 107–108, 110, 121
psychosynthesis, cosmic, 23
psychotherapy, 219
psyllium seeds, 237
purging and cleansing, 131, 248

quartz, as healing stone, 11, 104
Quenched Wine, 240–241

recipes
  Creamed Spelt Soup, 104
  Fennel Eye Remedy, 76
  Fennel Tea, 76
  Good as Gold, 93
  Lily Oil, 75
  Parsley-Honey Wine, 249
  Pear Honey, 101–102
  Quenched Wine, 241
  Rose-Sage Oil, 75
  Sage Tea, 135
  Spice Cookies for the Nerves, 238
  Vegetable-Spelt Broth, 248
  Violet Elixir, 242
relationships, importance of, 43
remembering, 180–181
remorse, as virtue, 6, 40, 192–197
repentence, 229
reverence, as virtue, 7, 40, 212–215
reverence for God, as virtue, 5, 40, 149–153
rock crystal water, 104
Rose-Sage Oil, 75
ruby, as healing stone, 160
rue, 242, 243

Sage Tea, 135
salvation, as virtue, 4, 40
sapphire
  as healing stone, 112, 156
  as wine, 164
sardonyx
  as healing stone, 153, 197
  as strengthener of the senses, 238
satisfaction, as virtue, 7, 40, 225–230
saved soul, as virtue, 133–136
savory, 240
scurrility, as vice, 7, 40, 212–215
self-analysis, 43–44
senses, five, 48
senses, seven, in the east, 61–62
seraphim, role of, in healing, 50
seven
  childhood virtues, 137–139
  deeds of compassion, 82–87
  number, significance of, 22, 25, 37
  powers (east), 60–62
sexuality, 164–165
skin diseases, 91
smell. *See also* aromatherapy
  role of, in healing, 49, 75–79
  and oats, 239
smoking, fasting to quit, 247
soul
  capacities of, 21–22
  healing power of, 29–30, 58–59
  and life energy, 23–24
  power center of, 183–184

relationship with body, 22, 24–33
three forces of, 30–31
sound
of the earth, 147–148
of the sun, 148
speech, role of, in healing, 49
spelt, 83, 102, 237
as part of fast, 244–250
Spice Cookies for the Nerves, 238
spirituality, loss of, 235
stability, as virtue, 6, 7, 40, 185–188, 215–218
stones, healing. *See* crystals and stones
stress, and fasting, 245
suicide, 235
sun, sound of, 148
symbols, visionary, 3–7, 8–9

taste, role of, in healing, 49
tetragrammaton, 18
thirst for glory, as vice, 5, 40, 149–153
three
forces of love, 145
number, significance of, 25
touch, role of, in healing, 49
tranquillity, as virtue, 3, 40, 92–103
Trinity, 10, 33–37, 159, 204
truth, as virtue, 4, 40, 117–121
turbulenta materia, 204
twelve, number, significance of, 36

unhappiness, as vice, 4, 40, 124–128

vagabondage, as vice, 7, 40, 215–218
Vegetable-Spelt Broth, 248
vegetarians and cancer, 111
vertebrae
and connection to organs, 2, 3–7
and connection to virtues and vices, 3–7, 42
vices. *See* virtues and vices
Violet Elixir, 242
viriditas, 15, 124, 133, 149, 164–165, 168, 247
virtues and vices, 3–7, 39–43, 43–44, 48
body and relation to, 54, 56–58
childhood, 137–139
in the east (1–7), 60–106
and elders (31–35), 208–243
in the north (16–22), 137–167
in the south (23–30), 168–207
in the west (8–15), 107–136
visionary symbols, 3–7, 8–9
vita activa, 132
vita contemplativa, 132
vitamin and mineral supplements, 100, 102
vortex energy, 152, 204

wars against evil, 171–172
water, and compassion, 83–84
Weltschmerz, 230–231, 235
wickedness, as vice, 4, 40, 115–117
wife, value of, 178
will, as power in the soul, 30–31
wine as therapy
gold topaz, 62
onyx, 104
parsley-honeywine, 106
quenched, 240–241
wisdom, 169–170
women, role of, 28

yearning for God, as virtue, 3, 40, 103–106

About Hildegard of Bingen

Hildegard was born in 1098 in Bermersheim, near Alzey, in Rhine Hessen, Germany. According to the custom of the Middle Ages, she—the tenth child—was handed over to God's care as a tithe and consequently grew up in the cloister at Disibodenberg. There, her sisters of the Order of Saint Benedict unanimously voted her abbess. Ever since childhood she possessed a special charisma, the gift of vision, which connected her with universal wisdom. As the abbess Hildegard studied and gained an understanding of all the secrets of the cosmos. She wrote visionary works in theology, music, medicine, and what we today call psychotherapy. In her medicine Hildegard emphatically points out the connections among body, soul, and mind. In her work she describes the healing powers hidden in nature and gives instructions on how to treat and care for the body holistically. Hildegard of Bingen died in the year 1189, at the age of eighty-one.

About the Author

Wighard Strehlow, Ph.D., was born on September 22, 1939, in Stettin, Germany. He studied natural sciences at the Technical University in Berlin and received a post-doctoral fellowship to Yale University. He then gained thirteen years of chemical research experience in the pharmaceutical industry. In 1980 he received training and official certification in nontraditional medicine. Since 1984, he has been the successor to Dr. Gottfried Hertzka in the Hildegard practice in Konstanz, Germany.